Richard L Blake DPM MS

PRACTICAL
BIOMECHANICS

FOR The PODIATRIST

BOOK 3:

MECHANICAL CHANGES COMMON FOR VARIOUS INJURIES
(ANKLE AND ABOVE)
VARIOUS CONCEPTS AND THEIR ROLE IN TREATMENT
PRONATION AND SUPINATION SYNDROMES
LIMB LENGTH DISCREPANCY
WEAK AND TIGHT MUSCLES
POOR SHOCK ABSORPTION AND VARIOUS INSTABILITIES

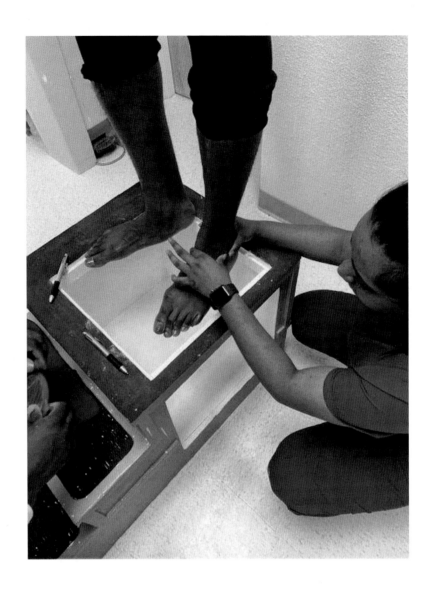

Practical Biomechanics for the Podiatrist
Book 3

By

Richard L Blake DPM MS

Past President, American Academy of Podiatric Sports Medicine
Adjunct Faculty, California School of Podiatric Medicine
42 Years Podiatrist at Sports and Orthopedic Institute
Saint Francis Memorial Hospital, San Francisco, California

The medical information contained in this book, including treatment and/or product recommendations, are solely the opinion of the author.

ISBN 979-8-35091-696-6

Book Baby Publishing

7905 N Crescent Blvd

Pennsauken, NJ, 08110

Introduction

Welcome to the 4 Book Series entitled: Practical Biomechanics for the Podiatrist.These books represent my life's work in the field of biomechanics, podiatry, and sports medicine. And, these fields are continuing to grow. I have tried to learn from everyone, as there are hidden truths in every theory and every treatment modality. You also have to help your patients first and foremost, and each patient comes in with individual ideas that will greatly affect your treatment. This therefore represents my relationship to my patients based on science, respect, and humility. I hope the pages represent me well.

The 4 books will be published in order, and finished next year 2024. Book 1 and 2 came out last year, 2022. The Table of Contents on the book's back covers all 4 books so that the reader can see what is coming next. Thank you for joining me on my journey helping treat my patients with love. Biomechanics has been an incredible cornerstone to that journey and I thank all the fine teachers I had in this field.

I am so thrilled in this book to be helped by two Spanish Podiatrists: Carlos Martínez Sebastián and Álvaro Gómez Carrión. They expertly discuss various concepts in Chapter 8 all Podiatrists should be aware of. They have already translated 2 of my previous books into Spanish. I am very thankful to Dr Joseph D'Amico who is preparing a chapter for the next book and wrote the Foreword to Book 1. I am so thankful to Dr Timothy Dutra for writing the Foreword to this book. Dr Dutra and I share our passions for biomechanics and teaching. We are both Past Presidents of the American Academy of Podiatric Sports Medicine. He works full time teaching biomechanics at the California School of Podiatric Medicine in Oakland, California.

This book is really about layers.In medicine, layers can represent various treatment approaches when one approach is not successful. I am hopeful that this book series gets you past protocols to injuries to more individual approaches to successful treatments. We all need our starting points, but true mastery of this art of medicine requires going deeper. I will close with this wonderful quote from Ralph Waldo Emerson. I hope this book with your next step, and be the individual Mr Emerson is describing.

"All great masters are chiefly distinguished by the power of adding a second, third, and perhaps a fourth step in a continuous line. Many a man had taken the first step. With every additional step you enhance immensely the value of your first."

Dedication

I would love to dedicate this book to my students at the California School of Podiatric Medicine, Samuel Merritt University, Oakland, California. As volunteer faculty, I spend time with the 2nd and 3rd Year Students. Year after year, their lively spirits and curious minds motivate me. They have become my muse for my writing. I want them to begin where I am ending my career in both knowledge and wisdom, and take off from there. There is so much more to be learned in the 3 main fields that this book touches upon: Podiatry, Sports Medicine, and Biomechanics. It is my hope that my students, and students from all the Podiatry schools across the globe, take the present knowledge and expand on it. Both you and the profession are at a beginning point only in our knowledge. There is so much more to learn.

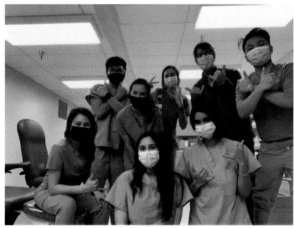 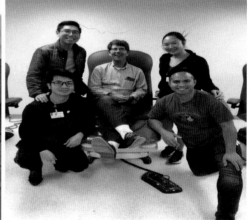

My direct message to podiatry students:

For the students that I have personally taught, thank you for your gift of keeping me young, curious, and invigorated. You will never regret joining the wonderful healing profession of Podiatry. Always find the fun in what you are doing through what brings you joy. When patients are not getting better, develop Plan B. Know that your help with your patients can be the most important contribution to their health, even for problems above the foot and ankle. So, keep learning, find your own truths in medicine, don't let protocols always dictate what you do, and schedule your practice so you can heal your patients routinely with your time, good spirit, and a smile. Listen to your patients for every word they say can be important, and learn to love your patients as it will bring you peace. You have joined the healing arts. Podiatry's role in the health of our nation and world is vital. Thank you for deciding to join this healing work.

Table of Contents (Book 3)

Foreword

by Timothy Dutra DPM, MS, MHCA

Assistant Professor, Samuel Merritt University College of Podiatric Medicine
Podiatric Team Physician, Intercollegiate Athletics, University of California, Berkeley
Clinical Director, Special Olympics Northern California Healthy Athletes Fit Feet Program
Past President & Fellow, American Academy of Podiatric Sports Medicine
Diplomate, American Board of Podiatric Medicine/ CAQ Podiatric Sports Medicine
Diplomate, American Board of Medical Specialties in Podiatry, Podiatric Sports Medicine
Past Vice-Chair & Board of Directors, Joint Commission on Sports Medicine & Science
Distinguished Practitioner, National Academies of Practice/ Fellow, Podiatric Medicine Academy
Fellow, American College of Sports Medicine
Fellow, American College of Podiatric Medicine

It is a great honor and privilege to write the foreward for Practical Biomechanics for Podiatrist Volume 3 of a four volume series. There is a great need for a practical biomechanics book series for students, residents, and practitioners for learning, reviewing, refreshing their skill base, and keeping up with the developing treatment options for their patients. Our biomechanics faculty at the college stress to our podiatry students that biomechanics is the foundation of our profession, and understanding concepts can be challenging but essential to a good patient outcome.

I am so thankful that Dr. Blake has taken on the tremendous task of writing this four volume series of Practical Biomechanics and making it understandable, practical, and valuable for our everyday treatment of our active patients.

This is a well-written, concise book covering a wealth of clinical information. The knowledge can be applied daily in practice to include a comprehensive and individual treatment plan covering all bases. The practical biomechanics questions in each section provide for a great review of the topics covered in this volume. It is very comprehensive in its coverage and addresses mechanical changes that influence injuries. Dr. Blake does a very good job of discussing orthotic prescription and modifications, training techniques, taping, bracing, shoe modifications, muscle strengthening and stretching exercises, rehabilitation, pain management, and return to activity suggestions.

I have had the pleasure of working with Dr. Blake throughout my podiatric career, beginning as a student at the California College of Podiatric Medicine with Dr. Blake teaching in our biomechanics and sports medicine classes, as well as covering orthotic prescription, fabrication, and adjustments. Like many of our former podiatry students, biomechanics and sports medicine was the primary force for pursuing a career in podiatric medicine and surgery. Biomechanics is the foundation of podiatry. The better we understand and apply biomechanics to our care and treatment of our patients, the better and more consistent the outcomes will be. I appreciated his passion, enthusiasm, and energy for the profession, as well as his love for teaching and education. I have gotten to know Rich as a colleague, practicing in the Bay Area, as well as through our involvement with the American Academy of Podiatric Sports Medicine. During the later phase of my career as a faculty member at Samuel Merritt University College of Podiatric Medicine, Dr. Blake has continued to work with our students in our biomechanics classes graciously and patiently sharing his knowledge and expertise with them. Our podiatry students appreciate the caring personality that Rich demonstrates with his patience in teaching skills, and his passion for understanding human movement and gait. Like Dr. Blake, I share the passion for biomechanics and sports medicine, which attracted many of us into a career in podiatry. Rich is one of the most humble, intelligent, and professional colleagues that I know, and he has served as one of my valuable mentors throughout my career in practice and academics.

Practical Biomechanics for Podiatrist Book 3 continues the series coverage in different aspects of biomechanics, and it includes chapters on Mechanical Changes Common for Various Injuries, Various Theories and Their Role in Treatment, Pronation and Supination Syndromes, Limb Length Discrepancy, Weak and Tight Muscles, and Poor Shock Absorption and Various Instabilities. I have always appreciated Dr. Blake's individually tailored treatment plans for approaching injuries and developing alternate plans if the injury is not improving satisfactorily for the expected time line and return to activity level. He stresses that we need to understand the mechanics of the problem presented by our patients so that we can better deal with cause, cause reversal, and treatment options. The treatment plan is a contract between the treating physician and patient, so that the goals and objectives are common, as well as understanding the biomechanics and cause of the injury and what is needed to help heal and prevent further problems.

Having come from a kinesiology and athletic training background, I have always appreciated Dr. Blake's' approach to gait evaluation (checklist) by looking at the entire process from head to toe, assessing symmetry, compensation, weak links, etc. Dr. Blake's' philosophies such as the KISS principle (keep it simple stupid), rule of three (most overuse injuries are caused by at least three factors); Occam's razor (the simplest solution to a problem is most likely the case), etc. are all helpful to review for both students and practitioners alike. The importance of pain management, sport specific rehabilitation/cross training methods, as well as return to activity guidelines are very helpful to understanding and treating the specific injuries. Dr. Blake is passing on his passion and enthusiasm for biomechanics and the profession of podiatry, and I am very grateful for his energy and love of teaching our podiatry students and practitioners.

Enjoy and continue to learn the joy of biomechanics in your practice! This four volume series is a valuable addition to your professional reference library for a timely review of material and practical biomechanics questions to help reinforce and build your biomechanics foundation.

Much of my teaching philosophy is influenced by Dr. Blake's academic teaching and clinical approach, along with biomechanics faculty at CCPM, including Dr. Ronald Valmassy, Dr. Paul Scherer, Dr. Kevin Kirby, Dr. Chris Smith, followed by Dr. Doug Richie and Dr. John Pagliano during my postgraduate residency and podiatric sports medicine fellowship. I consider myself a child of the American Academy of Podiatric Sports Medicine family, as I founded the first student chapter while a student at CCPM, completed an AAPSM Fellowship in Training Program with Dr John Pagliano in Long Beach, California, became a Fellow, became a board member and President, served as an Advisor for the SMUCPM Student Chapter of the AAPSM, served in mentor program, and volunteered with Special Olympics as Clinical Director. I also owe a huge debt of gratitude to the late Dr Bill Olson, who recruited me to help teach the sports medicine class at CCPM, and later assisted getting me on as Podiatric Team Physician with Cal Sports over 20+ years ago, and mentoring me with collegiate athletics covering 30 different sports teams at Cal. Bill had that passion for sports medicine and teaching the sports medicine interns and athletic trainers, giving frequent in-services and presentations to the athletic training staff. Podiatric sports medicine became much more than teaching runners, but covering all the other sports. I was very fortunate that this group of mentors all stressed the importance of understanding the influence of biomechanics on treatment outcome and recovering from injury, as well as minimizing re-injury or additional injuries in the future.

Chapter 7: Mechanical Changes Common for Various Injuries (Ankle and Above)

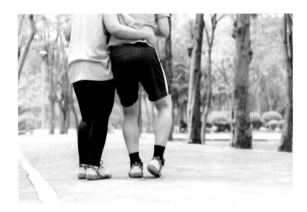

The Injured Ankle

I am so hopeful that these lists will help you experiment to find the solution for the pain your patients suffer. What works for one patient, may or may not work for another. What works for the right foot, in cases of bilateral pain, may not work for the left foot. Mechanical changes sometimes need to be additive, therefore it can take 3 or 4 mechanical changes to help the most. With each visit, unless you are maintaining 0-2 pain levels, as you progress your patients through the phases of rehabilitation, keep experimenting to find out what works to maintain that level of pain often considered "Good Pain" or pain that will not prevent the overall healing. Many patients have stopped previous successful treatments because they did not help completely. I find the additive approach of 4-5 treatments can be very successful, even if one individual treatment was only 20% helpful by itself.

Practical Biomechanics Question #324: What are the 3 Phases of Rehabilitation? What Phase typically uses casts? What Phase typically begins a Walk/Run Program? (Answer: 689)

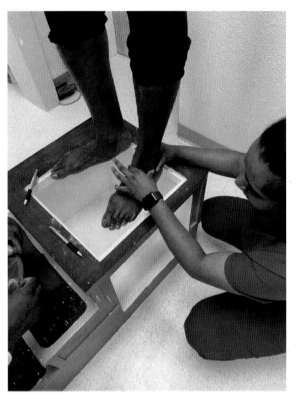

Podiatry Students in my class at the California School of Podiatric Medicine assessing the foot and leg structure of patients

What is the role of Podiatrists in the 2020s and beyond from the knee up? This Chapter 7 firmly discusses our role. I tell my podiatry students that their contribution to a patient's knee, hip, or low back problem may be the most important of all the health care providers. Some Podiatrists with a good sports medicine practice routinely deal with runner's knees, hip, and chronic low back pain. Runner's come in with their plantar fasciitis, achilles and shin splints, but will also be complaining of knee, hip or back problems. As you treat the foot and ankle, you find that other problems can get better. Where other Podiatrists are sort of forced into knowing the foot hip or foot knee or foot low back relationship. A treatment may help the foot, but irritate the knee. The treatment for foot pain helps some for the foot, but miraculously for the patient's back, hip or knee. The more you understand about the overall leg biomechanics (see Chapters 3 and 4 particularly), the more you will begin to understand why any change (for better or worse) happens. And, you will begin to predict these changes and the successful treatments for the patient's benefit.

Anterior Ankle Impingement Syndrome

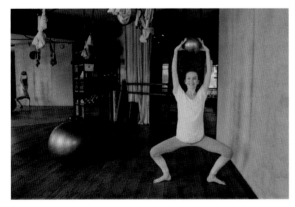

The Deep Plie Position in Ballet potentially jams the front of the ankle causing anterior ankle impingement syndrome

Anterior Ankle Impingement Syndrome is typically a combination of bony and soft tissue issues. One of the mistakes made is to see a large anterior tibial spur or dorsal talar spur, combined with the symptoms that present, and immediately think of surgery as the only cure.

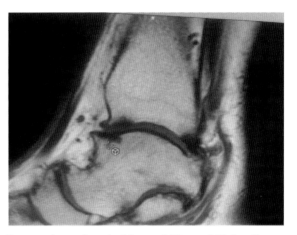

Large Anterior Ankle and Dorsal Talar Spur causing Anterior Ankle Joint Impingement Symptoms

Most of the time the symptoms can be calmed down, and with a careful maintenance program, the patient is allowed back to their normal activities. I explain to patients that if we see a spur we have to assume that it has been there for years. I ask myself why is it hurting now and can it be calmed down? This being said, a large spur may need surgery, and I discuss with my patients that they should see a surgeon to know about what would be done if it came down to surgery. This is my approach to any patient that may need surgery while I am conservatively trying to avoid surgery. Most of the time, they present back to me with greater vigor or commitment to attempt to avoid surgery. Of course, besides these mechanical discussions below, anti-inflammatory measures are also being used at the same time. Typically, these joints will have some degenerative joint disease, so I really try to minimize cortisone shots which can stop the normal healing process.

Practical Biomechanics Question #325: Why would heel lifts help patients with anterior ankle impingement? (A. 689)

Practical Biomechanics Question #326: Why would a weak achilles tendon cause anterior ankle impingement pain? (A. 689)

To tie this into Chapter 3 and 4 on gait and biomechanical examination (Books 1 and 2 respectively), with anterior ankle pain we are looking for signs of supination which can cause compression forces at the medial border of the joint, or pronatory signs that maybe indicate excessive torque across the ankle, or very weak achilles tendons which would not protect the anterior ankle joint, or boney blocks to ankle dorsiflexion, and the most important examinations to do in 10 minutes (or 20 minutes) are:

- RCSP (for pronation or supination)
- Ankle Joint Dorsiflexion (for osseous equinus or hypermobility) including Lunge Test
- Single Heel Raise (for achilles strength)
- Ligamentous Laxity tests of Push-Pull, Varus Stress, Transverse Translation
- Pes Cavus Foot Type on observation with its natural crowding of the front

of the ankle due to the high calcaneal inclination angle

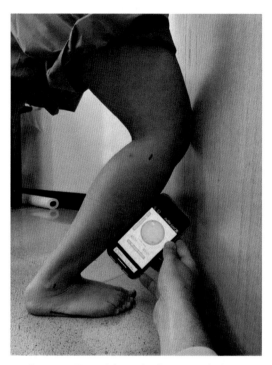

Lunge Test (description Book 2 pages 201-2) showing over flexibility of the Achilles tendon and too much compression on the anterior aspect of the ankle joint

Common Mechanical Changes for Anterior Ankle Impingement Syndrome (with the common ones used in RED)
1. Heel Lifts
2. Heeled Shoes
3. Avoidance of Zero Drop Shoes
4. 2 Positional Single Leg Heel Raises
5. Extensor Tendon Stretching
6. Talar Mobilization
7. Single Leg Balancing
8. Avoidance of Fully Dorsiflexed Ankle Positions
9. Eliminate Any Lateral Instability
10. Avoidance of Negative Heel Positions
11. Creating Pronation When Needed
12. Achilles Tendon Taping

13. Training Techniques
14. Correcting Soleus Weakness

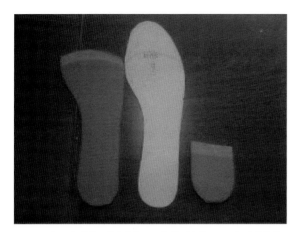

Here both Heel Lift and Full Length Lift is Demonstrated

Heel Lifts are the most common and simple mechanical change we can make with anterior ankle impingement syndrome. The mechanical function is to take pressure off the front of the ankle by slightly plantar flexing the ankle. Many of us have abused our ankles and now have anterior bone spurs. Some of us just have shallow ankle joints with not a lot of clearance anteriorly, or weak achilles that allow our ankles to bend forward too much in dorsiflexion. In these cases the front of the ankles can get irritated. Heel lifts are the perfect fix, in fact they can be glued right to the orthotic device if the patient already has them. When you need a heel lift only on one side for this problem, and you are not sure if that is the short leg, you should put the same amount of lift on the other side for balance. Heel lifts are normally made out of rubber or a cork and rubber composite. I typically use ¼ inch heel lifts that I make out of sheets of rubber cork from JMS Plastics.
https://jmsplastics.com/product/rubber-cork/

An initial visit recommendation of heel lifts (dispensed) and ice pack for 20 minutes 3 times a day can immediately get the patient moving in the right direction and follows the KISS principle. The Occam's Law of Anterior Ankle Impingement Syndrome is to Always Use Heel Lifts.

Practical Biomechanics Question #327: Explain why heel lifts work in anterior ankle impingement syndrome? (A. 689)

Heeled Shoes can help anterior ankle impingement, while the soft tissue is getting calmed down, better than heel lifts or removable boots. The mechanical function is also to take pressure off the front of the ankle by slightly plantar flexing the ankle. Up to 2 inch heels can be needed to clear the front of the ankle as you go through dorsiflexion in gait mainly during midstance. Of course, the selection of such shoes, even for a 4 hour period of each day, is easier for women than men. Some athletic shoes are ½ inch already, and when you add an additional ½ inch as a heel lift, you are easily getting enough push forward for normal push off. Around the house, patients can use Dansko clogs with a 2 inch heel height to help free up the front of the ankle, or the daily use of Elevator Shoes from TallMenShoes.com for men. Women do have a world of more choices.
https://www.tallmenshoes.com/

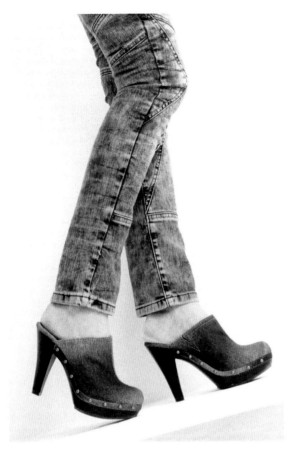

Clog used for anterior ankle impingement

Practical Biomechanics Question #328: Tallmenshoes.com can add 3 inches to men's height. When would you use this for anterior ankle impingement syndrome?(689)

Avoidance of Zero Drop Shoes is crucial for at least the initial stages of anterior ankle impingement. The mechanical function is to prevent the excessive crowding of the front of the ankle during midstance. Every 1/16 inch of heel height from both shoes and inserts can make a difference. As the inflammation dies down, even in the presence of spur formation, hopefully you can lower this restriction as long as other conservative measures are maintained.

Practical Biomechanics Question #329: What crowds the front of the ankle more–traditional running shoes or zero drop shoes like Altras? (Answer: 689)

2 Positional Single Leg Heel Raises are crucial for not only maintaining, but improving, great achilles strength. 2 positional means that the exercise is done in 2 positions. In this case, the heel raises are done with the knee both straight and bent. The mechanical function is to add posterior resistance to the forward motion of the tibia which can crowd the front of the ankle. The stronger your achilles, both gastrocnemius and soleus, the easier you can avoid collapsing the midfoot, jamming up the anterior ankle, and prolonging pronation into the propulsion. When you have a good achilles, your tendon will fire at the right time plantarflexing your ankle appropriately. This can get confused with equinus when the tight muscles increase pronation, and can increase the jamming of the anterior ankle. These are the cases where the athlete or patient was allowed to get strong while not keeping their good flexibility. When you get stronger but tighter, you have to stay with a normal range of flexibility or something will happen negatively. By 2 positional single leg heel raises, I am talking about slowly going up and down with the heel, each side separately, trying to build up to 25 straight knee and 12-15 bent knee. With a patient fairly weak, first they build up to 50 two sided heel raises knee straight, and 25 two sided heel raises with knee bent. Slowly they begin to add single sided ones and take away from the two sided ones. It can be a

6-12 month progression with the provider helping them maintain flexibility. This process will be explained in more detail in Chapter 11 of this book.

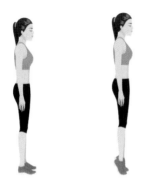

2 Sided Gastrocnemius (knee straight) heel raises are demonstrated

Extensor Tendon Stretching is typically crucial in pes cavus feet. The tighter the extensors, the more the ankle joint is anteriorly jammed. The mechanical function is to allow the ankle to plantar flex easing the tension in the front of the ankle. Stretching by sitting on top of our feet is usually too painful and causes the tissue to tighten up more. I love one of the modified quadricep stretches where you place the tops of your toes on the edge of a table behind you. The quadriceps are also getting stretched as the leg that is standing goes deeper into a squat to feel the pull in the front of the ankle. This is typically a 30 second stretch done 3 times daily.

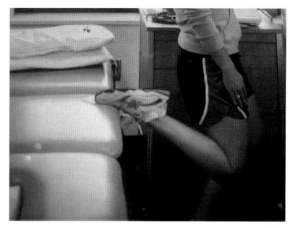

Extensor tendon stretching demonstrated as a modified Quadriceps stretch

Practical Biomechanics Question #330: Explain why stretching the foot extensors can ease stress in the front of the ankle joint. (Answer: 689)

Talar Mobilization is usually the work of a manual physical therapist or foot chiropractor, although podiatrists like Drs Howard Dananberg or Timothy Shea are experts. The mechanical function of talar mobilization is not to create more than normal motion, but to unstick a talus jammed into a certain spot. That spot in my practice tends to me anterior and medial. When there is less motion due to this dysfunction of the talus, stress and pain occurs. Freeing up a"stuck" talus so it glides easier can greatly help these symptoms. If you send a patient to Physical Therapy for anterior ankle impingement syndrome, see if they feel that the talus is jammed somehow and needs to be freed up.

Practical Biomechanics Question #331: Mobilization techniques are Graded 1-5. What Grade would you do when there is a lot of pain in the ankle, and what grade would you do with no pain in the ankle? 689

Single Leg Balancing is a simple, powerful, functional exercise to tone up the ankle. The mechanical function is to strengthen the entire ankle to decrease any instability that can irritate the ankle. I feel it is a great diagnostic test for overall functional ankle strength. The weaker the patient is, the more they collapse into the arch early on in their daily exercises with the talus medially deviated. The stronger the patient is, the more they will move over the ankle correctly. I have the patients perform this with shoes on or off when they remember it in the evening. Get in a doorway so they can catch themselves as they balance 2 minutes on each foot. Slowly they will not have to hold on to the door well at all during the 2 minutes. After they accomplish that they can begin to add time with their eyes closed, or attempt to stand in the middle of a soft pillow.

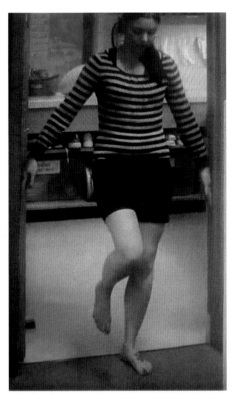

Single Leg Balancing with help from the Door Well

Avoidance of Fully Dorsiflexed Ankle Positions is important especially as you are trying to calm the anterior ankle impingement with localized synovitis down. Its mechanical function is to prevent overload to the front of the ankle. The ankle is the most crowded anteriorly with the ankle dorsiflexed and the knee bent. In this position, you have lost the protective function of the gastrocnemius and the ankle bend can pinch the bones or soft tissue in front of the ankle. You have to review with your patients the activities that they are doing. Lunges are typically okay, but not squats for example. Several of many yoga poses may be off limits for a while. Stiff uphill climbs will also crowd the front of the ankle if the patient can not stay on their toes. A simple history of what the patient is doing, and usually a few restrictions will get them thinking about these biomechanics. Most of my patients come back into the office for their followup visit excited to tell me other actions that they were doing that were crowding the front of the ankle that they now were trying to avoid.

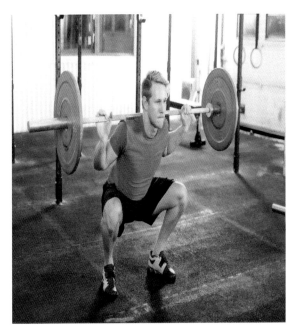

Weight lifter in full dorsiflexed position crowding the anterior ankle

Practical Biomechanics Question #332: Would plie or releve in ballet irritate the anterior ankle in anterior ankle impingement syndrome? (Answer: 689)

Eliminating any Lateral Instability is crucial since over supination causes the medial aspect of the talus to jam upwards into the tibia. The mechanical function of eliminating lateral instability (also called contact phase subtalar joint supination) is to prevent the medial talar dome from impinging into the distal medial tibia. The patient may or may not be able to tell you

where the impingement occurs, such as medial or just in the front of the ankle. This is worse in pes cavus that are laterally unstable (seen in almost one third of all pes cavus feet walking barefoot, and even more when they wear unstable shoes). As we have talked on changing mechanical forces with simple to complex methods (Book 2 Chapter 5), I will list in Chapter 13 (Book 4) on custom made orthotic devices all of the RX variables that help control over supination tendencies.

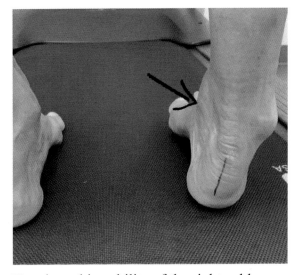

Here lateral instability of the right ankle stretches the lateral side of the foot and ankle and impinges the medial side

Practical Biomechanics Question #333: Which of the following is not for correcting lateral instability. There can be more than one answer. (Answer: 689)
1. Deep Heel Cups
2. Denton Modification
3. Valgus Wedging
4. Kirby Skives (medial or lateral)
5. Rearfoot post motion
6. Forefoot Varus Support

Avoidance of Negative Heel Positions is really an aspect of avoiding fully dorsiflexed positions to its extreme. The mechanical function is to minimize the anterior impingement of the ankle joint. I am talking of the practice of lowering your heel below the plane of the metatarsals with your heel not supported (and therefore your rearfoot is not protected). When the ankle is placed in this vulnerable position, with 50 to 100% of body weight on top of it, not only does the front of the ankle get potentially beat up, but so does the achilles, plantar fascia, long plantar ligament, and spring ligament. It is really the standing negative heel that has seemed to injure my athletes in the past. Similar positions seen in walking uphills with the back foot, or doing a downward dog in Yoga, seems much less stressful.

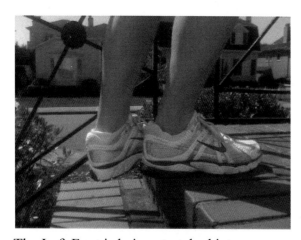

The Left Foot is being stretched into a Negative Heel Position where the heel is below the plane of the forefoot

Practical Biomechanics Question #334: When you compare the heel to ball relationship during a prolonged downward dog to standing achilles stretch with the heel dropped off a platform, what in terms of body weight stress or force moments are different between these two exercises? (689)

Creating Pronation When Needed is the essential task we need to do in patients with rigid feet typically having pes cavus, or laterally unstable patients at heel strike we just talked about. The mechanical function is to create the needed contact phase pronation of the subtalar joint vital in lower extremity motion. This is because contact phase subtalar joint pronation is crucial and the talus is going to move and adapt to the ground. The talus will plantar flex on the tibia at foot strike, but to avoid being jammed into the ankle joint mortise with ankle joint dorsiflexion, the subtalar and midtarsal joints must be pronating. Therefore, some orthotic devices just have to have 4 degrees of pronation motion placed into the rearfoot post to create pronation, while others need to first stop contact phase subtalar joint supination, and then encourage subtalar joint pronation.

Achilles Tendon Taping is another method besides heel heights to help the ankle plantar flex and avoid excessive anterior jamming. Its mechanical function is to slow down the ankle dorsiflexion that jams the anterior ankle joint. Taping is never a long term solution like heel lifts can be, but can help in activities that the patient may bend their ankle too much. Commonly I use achilles taping both during the short term rehabilitation of an acute episode, always along with heel lifts, while they are icing, etc. But, in cases of potential surgery like a dorsal talar spur, I may use the taping as long term prevention.

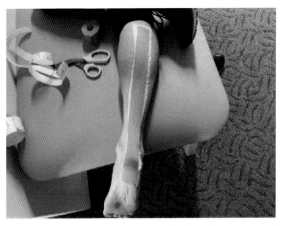

Achilles Tendon Taping with Leukotape and Coverall

Practical Biomechanics Question #335: When taping the achilles tendon, is the goal to limit the ankle bend completely? (A:689)

Training Techniques may be something you just impart to the physical therapist, athletic trainer, or coach working with you, but it is crucial that you understand. The mechanical function is to allow excessive compression force on the front of the ankle. This aspect of treating a patient can undermine all the work you are doing if not properly addressed. If you treat ballet dancers with anterior ankle impingement, they can do all the pointe work they want, but you have to have them avoid plies for a while until you really get their symptoms under control. For runners, you advise them to stay off running uphills unless they can stay on their toes. For football, rugby, etc. they will be out of action for a while due to the severe ankle bend which is part of every activity. If the athlete crosstrains with a stationary bike, have them raise the seat higher than normal to avoid crowding the front of the ankle. These are all examples to give your patients to help get the idea across.

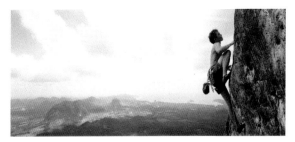

Rock Climbing is notorious for the athletes to get joints into excessive motions for prolonged time (here excessive ankle dorsiflexion and excessive knee flexion)

Correcting Soleus Weakness is one of my biggest challenges. Its mechanical function is to provide more posterior ankle protection when the knee is bent. I typically pick up soleus weakness when I measure for achilles tendon tightness. For anterior ankle impingement syndrome, the stronger the achilles (both gastrocnemius and soleus) is, the more protection to the front of the ankle. The converse is therefore true, the weaker the achilles tendon (both the gastrocnemius and soleus), the less protection to the front of the ankle. If the achilles is weak, and I find more cases of soleus weakness vs gastrocnemius weakness, the ankle will stay dorsiflexed much longer in the gait cycle, or just dorsiflex to a greater degree than with normal strength. The forward excursion of the tibia on the talus with a weak soleus or gastrocnemius is therefore longer, increasing the chance of soft tissue impingement of the anterior ankle. If you measure more than 15-18 degrees with the knee bent of ankle joint dorsiflexion, and my record is 36, you are dealing with a weak and over flexible soleus.

How can we also easily measure soleus strength? I take a very functional measurement when I ask the patient to perform heel raises in the office. First, I have them do 20 double sided heel raises to warm up. Then, I have them do max single heel raises with the knee extended (gastrocnemius strength). The gold standard is 25 for this which is equivalent to normal and good gastrocnemius strength. Then, I have them do max single leg heel raises with the knee bent (soleus strength). The gold standard is 12-13 for this which is equivalent to normal and good soleal strength.

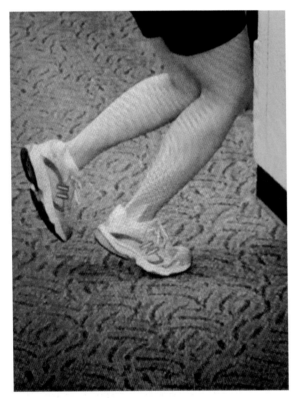

Here is bent knee single leg heel raises (also called calf raises) to strengthen the soleus

Practical Biomechanics Question #336: When a patient has anterior ankle impingement, what are the classic exercises to do? (Answer: 690)

Practical Biomechanics Question #337: When a ballet dancer began to get anterior ankle impingement symptoms, what positions (plie or releve) were immediately removed from practice? (Answer: 690)

Inversion Ankle Sprains

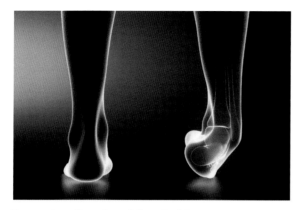

Inversion Sprain of the Ankle

We all treat an excessive number of inversion ankle sprains. It is one of the most common injuries, like plantar fasciitis, on this planet. Yet, there is a problem we must avoid in its familiarity. All ankle sprains are connected to very different people. We really have to individualize the mechanics and the needs of each patient to really help these patients. Ask yourself if the sprain was just bad luck, like a missed step, or are there predisposing factors at play (which of course could be that the patient is always in a hurry). If there are disposing factors, then these can be worked on and helped. Some of these predisposing factors are:

- Previous sprains
- Generalized ligamentous laxity
- Varus foot type (like rear foot varus)
- Forefoot Valgus/Plantarflexed first ray foot type
- Weak Peroneals
- Shoe Selection (including heels without heel stability)
- Activities which demand high lateral heel support

Previous ankle sprain(s), where the lateral ligaments are stretched out, is one of the mechanical reasons the ankle is functionally unstable. The adage that one ankle sprain leads to another ankle sprain comes from this instability and reluctance of athletes to treat their injuries seriously at times. Weak peroneal tendons can not protect the lateral ankle well, and can be a very successful treatment for chronic ankle instability. And, there are foot types, leg deformities, and athletic activities that put excessive stress on the lateral ankle and can be mitigated with recommendations and treatment.

Practical Biomechanics Question #338: When you think that a patient functions too inverted, especially with contact phase supination, what are 2 muscles to check for weakness? (Answer: 690)

To tie this into Chapter 3 and 4 on gait and biomechanical examination, in a patient recently experiencing an inversion ankle sprain, the most important examinations to do in 10 minutes (or 20 minutes) are:

- RCSP (to look for varus alignment)
- NCSP (to look for varus alignment)
- Ankle Ligament Stability tests
- Forefoot to Rearfoot Relationship (looking for everted forefoot deformities like plantar flexed first ray or forefoot valgus or pronatus)
- Peroneal Strength (longus, brevis, and tertius)
- Ankle Joint Dorsiflexion (too tight can cause both over pronation sometimes and oversupination in propulsion sometimes---the oversupination bad for ankle sprains

Common Mechanical Changes for Inversion Ankle Sprains (with the common ones used in RED)

1. Peroneal strengthening of longus and brevis
2. J Strap with leukotape to control inversion
3. Ankle braces
4. Mid calf or below the knee cam walker if need to drive pain to 0-2
5. EvenUp
6. Crutches
7. Single leg balancing
8. Valgus Wedges
9. Custom Orthotic Devices

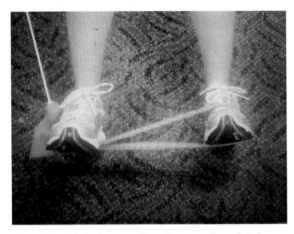

Theraband (a form of resistance bands) is used here to strengthen the left peroneus longus tendon (ankle at right angle and the patient goes sets of eversion repetitions)

Peroneal Strengthening of Longus and Brevis is crucial in stabilizing ankles and some Physical Therapists and Personal Trainers are good with this and some not. The mechanical function is to strengthen (thus stabilize) the lateral aspect of the ankle. The reason I mention that is that you should be good at this type of strengthening so you can evaluate what is going on. I always tell my patients that they can make

their ankles 3-4 times stronger pretty easily with some effort. Chapter 11 will be going through the progression of strength training from active range of motion to functional strength drills. It suffices to say that the peroneus longus is strengthened with the ankle at a right ankle and the foot everting. The peroneus brevis is strengthened when the ankle is plantar flexed and the foot everting.

Practical Biomechanics Question #339: What is the typical resistance band progression after 2 sets of 20 for both the peroneus longus and brevis tendons? (690)

J Strap with Leukotape to Control Inversion was previously explained with peroneal tendonitis problems (Chapter 6 Book 2). Its mechanical function is to decrease the supination moment on the lateral foot. This is typically used in the acute phase as the patient is weaning from the cam walker, or with a patient you sense has an unstable ankle pre or post sprain that needs more protection. I have had patients wear this tape at times when their ankle was more vulnerable for years, like hiking over rough trails. Leukotape can not be placed on the skin, so a product called Coverall is commonly sold together with it. Coverall is placed first to act as a skin protector.

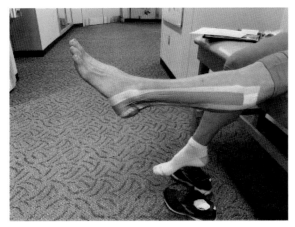

Leukotape for Inversion Resistance starts under the medial malleolus, goes under the heel, and up the lateral side of the foot

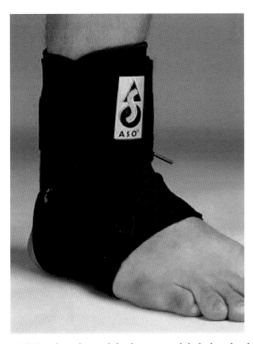

ASO classic ankle brace which both ties on and has re-enforcing velcro straps

Ankle Braces are an immediate protection, post cam walker, and can also be used for the long term. Their mechanical function is to stabilize the ankle and decrease stresses on the injured area. I have torn every ligament in my left ankle, so the protection of an ankle brace is nice for

sports like basketball with the lateral movements and the habit of landing on another's foot. All ankle braces pronate the subtalar joint of the patient, so perfect for inversion ankle sprains, but not perfect for all the ankle injuries I see patient's wearing them for like posterior tibial problems. I must highlight one of the traditional braces, the Aircast original, which protected side to side motions, but allowed the patient to move back to front.

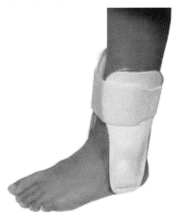

Aircast Original Stirrup Brace does not block sagittal plane motion

Practical Biomechanics Question #340: Would a low or high ankle sprain benefit the most from an Aircast Stirrup Brace and why? (Answer: 690)

Mid Calf and Below The Knee Cam Walker of course are the mechanical protection of an ankle sprain just after a sprain. Most Podiatrists stock them in their offices. Their mechanical function is to immobilize and rest the injured tissue to let healing begin. The height will depend on heel slippage with women needing the higher ones in general more often. Your heel can not be moving around in the boot if you are trying to protect it and calm the inflammation down. Depending on the severity of the injury, and whether any fractures also occurred, you could be in the walker for 2-3 months before you advance to a brace.

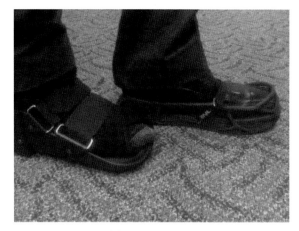

Here a Removable Boot (cam walker) is used on the injured right side and an EvenUp on the shoe of the left side

Practical Biomechanics Question #341: Why do patients with narrow heels need higher cam walkers? (Answer: 690)

EvenUp is a device that slips over the shoe on the side that does not have the cam walker to even the hip heights on both sides. The mechanical function is to even up the back when these boots are used for extended times. This is crucial for saving your back.

Crutches are necessary for moderate to severe ankle sprains. Their mechanical function in the initial days after an ankle sprain is to prevent the pain from getting out of control and to minimize the stress to the injured tissue. It is important to have the patient use crutches until full weight

bearing is comfortable and normal daily activities are achieved even with a boot or brace. With all injuries, I try to quickly get the patient to 0-2 pain level, and I have more success utilizing crutches up to the first month. Crutches should allow the patient to achieve a stable spine, and I never feel that they should advance from 2 crutches to one crutch. This will really hurt their back. It is either 2 crutches or no crutches is my mantra. Backpacks with crutches are the necessary way that a patient will carry their belongings even in my 80 year olds.

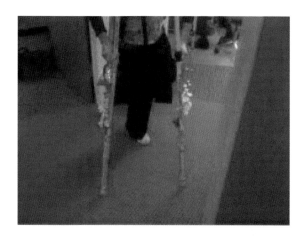

Practical Biomechanics Question #342: What is the chief difference between typical crutches and Canadian crutches? (A: 690)

Single Leg Balancing is both a strength and balance exercise of the ankle, knee, hip and core. Its mechanical function is to begin the buildup of strength and proprioceptive awareness of the injured ankle. It is probably the most important exercise we can do for our lower extremities besides single heel raises. It is the mainstay of re-strengthening our ankles post sprain. It is a 2 minute exercise each evening standing in a door well. You always want to make it more challenging. I typically progress patients from floor balancing eyes open, standing in the middle soft pillow eyes open, standing on balance disc eyes open, to finally standing on the floor with eyes closed. This progression may take 6 months if the ankle was very unstable to start with.

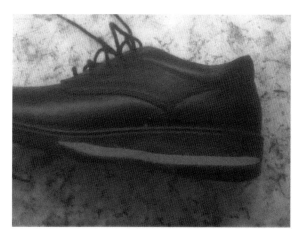

Midsole valgus wedge applied in the office only along part of the lateral side of the foot

Valgus Wedges can be simple ⅛ inch wedges added to shoe insoles to free standing heel or full foot wedges to midsole wedges up to ¼ inch to outsole wedges on some dress shoes. The mechanical function of the valgus wedge is to lessen the tendency to supinate. The goal of the wedges is to eliminate any lateral instability seen once gait evaluation can be done. The lateral instability can be so slight that the wedge is temporary, or so severe that wedging and special custom orthotic devices will eventually be made. One of the main thoughts I have with an ankle sprain patient is now to prevent the next one. And, since it will take awhile to get the patient super strong (my main goal), I need the

tricks of wedges, braces, taping, and stable shoes in the short term.

Practical Biomechanics Question #343: When applying a valgus wedge to a shoe, you have to watch a patient walk with the shoes on. What motion are you trying to prevent? (Answer: 690)

Custom Orthotic Devices will be mainly explored in Chapter 13 Book 4, but it is important to emphasize that you should have 3-4 orthotic devices that you can use for mild to severe overpronation, and 2-3 orthotic devices that you can use for mild to severe oversupination. The mechanical function of custom orthotic devices for ankle sprains is to prevent the ankle against lateral instability. The video link attached discusses the components of a custom orthotic device for patients that are laterally unstable. https://youtu.be/hMhrTmWXfDA

Practical Biomechanics Question #344: Name 6 common orthotic prescription components that can be used in lateral instability patients. (Answer: 690)

Ankle Instability

Ankle Instability is a problem with a certain level of surgical intervention so the stakes are high for conservative treatment to be successful. We are talking about instability of the lateral or outside of your ankle. Remember, the same treatments you are using to prevent surgery, will be important post surgery if required. There are 2 types of ankle instability, with one of them being the most important to the patient, and it is very important to differentiate. The 2 types of ankle instability are mechanical and functional. Mechanical instability means that there are mechanical positives to the tests you perform on the patient documenting that the ligaments are injured. These tests are varus stress (calcaneofibular ligament), or anterior posterior push pull (anterior talofibular ligament). There is also medial to lateral translation testing of subtalar joint instability. However, the most important type of instability is functional instability (where the patient does not trust their ankle). So many patients have mechanical instability, but no functional instability, or no mechanical instability (even in the face of previous ankle sprains) but significant functional instability, or both occurring at the same time. I therefore do not treat the test, or MRI, but the patient and try to find out why functional instability exists. It is functional instability that causes disability and must be eliminated.

To tie this into Chapter 3 and 4 on gait and biomechanical examination, with ankle instability, the most important examinations to do in 10 minutes (or 20 minutes) are:

- Generalized ligamentous laxity (like subtalar and midtarsal joint excessive range of motion)
- Positive ankle stability testing
- Single Leg Balancing
- Peroneal strength testing
- RCSP and NCSP (looking for varus conditions)
- Forefoot to Rearfoot Deformities (looking for causes of lateral instability like high forefoot valgus)
- Gait Evaluation noting Lateral Instability

Common Mechanical Changes for Ankle Instability (with the common ones used in RED)

1. Peroneal strengthening for longus and brevis
2. Proximal Muscle Strengthening and Positional Changes
3. Training Techniques
4. Single leg balancing
5. J Strap with leukotape to control inversion
6. Other Ankle Taping
7. Ankle Braces
8. Neutral shoes (not stability or motion control)
9. Avoiding Heels of Some Types
10. High Top Boots or AFOs
11. Prolotherapy

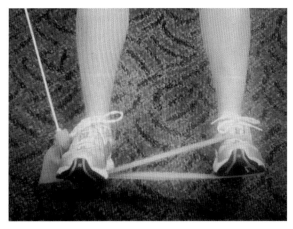

Strengthening of Peroneus Longus with the Ankle at a Right Angle to the Leg

Peroneal strengthening for longus and brevis is vital to stabilize the lateral side of the ankle. The mechanical function is to strengthen and support the lateral side of the ankle. Chapter 11 goes over the progression from simple to complex with strengthening. Strengthening is a graduated process as the patient gets stronger and stronger. The peroneus longus is strengthened by eversion of the ankle in a dorsiflexed position. The peroneus brevis is strengthened by eversion of the ankle in a plantarflexed or pointed position.

Practical Biomechanics Question #345: In an attempt to begin strengthening of the peroneal tendons, the patient started doing 2 sets of 10 repetitions Level 1 resistance bands in what 2 ankle positions? (A: 690)

Proximal Muscle Strengthening and Positional Changes can greatly protect the lateral ankle. The mechanical function is to assist in taking stress off the ankle in many ways. This was first shown in runners in the 1980s who would help their lateral ankles with less crossover in their gait (thus widened their base of gait). Now athletes of all sports can learn to cut (or laterally move) with their hips and not their ankles (perfected by Stephen Curry of the Golden State Warriors).

Proximal muscle strengthening refers to the hips and core. The stronger our legs are the less stress on the ankles and feet. Physical therapists refer to it as lifting the weight off your feet by strengthening the core and I like that imagery.

Training Techniques can be developed to put the least stress on the ankle. The mechanical function of this is to lessen the stress on the ankle and place it on the hip and core typically. The patient's base of gait can be widened doing certain drills, or the injured ankle is only stressed when wearing a brace. Trainers can remove repetitive drills that stress the ankle for other exercises of equal challenge.

Single leg balancing is mandated to everyone with bad ankles in my practice. It is a 2 minute single foot pose done in the evening to fatigue the ankle. The mechanical function is to both strengthen muscle/tendons, but wake up the neuromuscular connections for a reactive ankle responsive to slants, tilts, and cracks in the sidewalk. You need to always make it somewhat difficult or challenging by standing in shoes or barefoot, standing in the middle of a soft pillow or exercise disc, closing your eyes at times, or moving your hands with or without objects. The goal is to keep challenging yourself. The goal standard remains 2 minutes of single leg balancing with the eyes closed, yet only a few of my hearty patients get there.

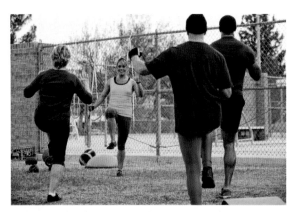

Every patient should have a single leg pose or exercise in their daily exercise regimen

Practical Biomechanics Question #346: Single Leg Balancing is a common exercise taught for ankle, knee, hip and low back rehabilitation. How long are these positions typically held? (Answer: 690)

J Strap with leukotape to control inversion has been previously described in peroneal tendonitis and inversion ankle sprains with a photo several pages ago. Its mechanical function is to decrease the stress on the lateral side of the ankle. It is used during at-risk activities that have the potential of developing a sprain like tennis, basketball, downhill hiking, etc.

Other Ankle Taping ranges from very restrictive, like a figure of 8 ankle lock, to slightly helpful (almost biofeedback quality) with some of the newer stretch tapes like Kinesio Tape, Kinesiology Technology Tape, RockTape, or Dynamic Tape. Their mechanical functions are to stabilize the lateral ankle but rarely to completely immobilize ankle inversion.

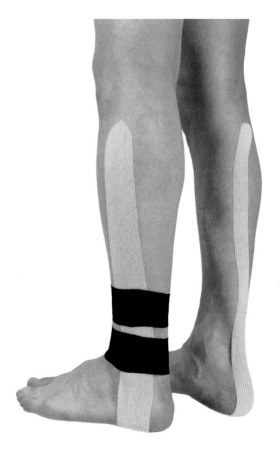

The left ankle here has one of the stretch tapes to support the lateral ankle without full restriction of motion

Ankle Braces need to block excessive inversion, but they tend to do either much more or hardly anything. Their mechanical function is to apply more or less resistance to inversion motion at a time when inversion of the foot and ankle should be restricted. I have always loved the traditional Aircast stirrup brace for varus instability (calcaneofibular ligament injuries) for its singularity of purpose. However, many of the anterior talofibular ligament tears need anterior support from tie-on braces like the ASO brace (Ankle Stabilizing Orthosis). There

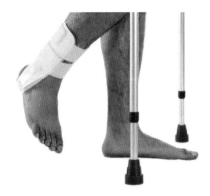

Aircast Stirrup Brace which blocks only Inversion

are so many incredible ankle braces to name here and providers tend to develop their favorites.

Practical Biomechanics Question #347: When addressing ankle instability, why would some patients only wear braces when playing sports? (Answer: 690)

Neutral shoes (not stability or motion control) are more important as the shoe breaks down. Their mechanical function is to ease medial weight shift in lateral ankle instability issues. You would hope the neutral shoe would pronate some when it began to break down, which is okay for lateral ankle instability. Motion control and stability shoes tend to be structured more medially leading to a varus lean as the shoe breaks down. This is very bad for lateral unstable patients. One of the points to make here is that ankle instability patients should have a visit when they bring all their shoes in to see if any are adding to the instability. Even when you point out lateral instability, aka excessive supination, many patients can

not feel the problem unless one side is so much worse than the other.

Avoiding Heels of Some Types is crucial for women with lateral instability, but only a general rule with many exceptions. The mechanical function is to allow the ankle to be more compressed in a dorsiflexed position and lower to the ground. Teach your patients to develop the sensation of when they are supinating. Contact phase supination is a terribly unstable motion and position to be in. They will learn to pick the heels that feel the most stable, usually with the wider heel platform "cuban".

ALL TYPES OF HEELS				
cone	cuban	italian	pin	wedge
flared	spool	stiletto	luigi XV	curved

Example of Various Heel Types with the Cuban Heel considered the most stable

High Top Boots or AFOs typically are worn in that order. Their mechanical function is to spread out the support to the lateral ankle up into the lower leg. As the patient feels more and more unstable, perhaps with repeated sprains, they will show up in your office with high top boots for that added protection. Or, in winter time, they may prefer the boots to a removable boot that would be dangerous outside for more acute injuries. It is in non-surgical patients, or patients being worked up for surgery, that AFOs can be helpful.

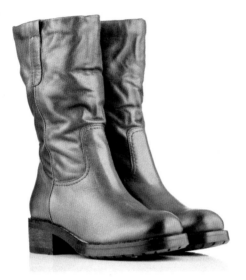

Here a form of high top boot is being used for extra ankle support

Practical Biomechanics Question #348: There are so many boots that can be worn year long if needed to help lateral ankle instability. What can you add to a boot to help lateral ankle problems? (Answer:690)

Prolotherapy is not a new or popular treatment in the podiatry world. Its mechanical function is to strengthen injured ligaments. It is the injection into ligaments of dextrose and water to irritate the ligament enough to cause some scarring. It is extremely beneficial for some to tighten their ligaments when overly stretched. I am not sure how it works if the ligament is completely torn. The EDS group of ligamentous laxity patients can get tremendous help from these simple injections. Its use is seeing a resurgence due to the popularity of regenerative medicine therapies.

Achilles Tendon Injuries

As we discuss achilles injuries, we need to discuss posterior heel pain, posterior ankle pain, and achilles tendon pain itself. There are alot of structures in the back of the ankle, so a definitive diagnosis can be hard to obtain initially. Patients come into the office with achilles pain primarily, or achilles pain secondary to something else. You examination should help differentiate, and always remember the achilles can hurt due to nerve pain from the low back (with a completely negative examination), or from compensation due to posterior heel bursitis or posterior ankle pathology.

Being into mechanics, my whole podiatric mindset is to keep the achilles strong and flexible and figure out what mechanics set up a situation where the strongest tendon in the body broke down. And, if the mechanics are not present, what am I missing? Perhaps the achilles is only sore due to its compensation for something else like os trigonum syndrome where the achilles is protecting the back of the ankle in an attempt to immobilize the tissue somewhat.

Practical Biomechanics Question #349: You could just focus your whole career on Achilles injuries; it is such an important structure. What are the 2 muscles that make up the achilles tendon? Answer: 691

The achilles tendon is the most powerful tendon in the body, and thus has a mighty great influence on the motions of the knee, ankle, and foot. Understanding the power it produces gives us the knowledge of the problems which happen when it does not function well.

Practical Biomechanics Question #350: We can gain so much information on the state of the achilles tendon by measuring its flexibility and strength. What does it mean when ankle joint dorsiflexion is 30 degrees with the knee extended in prone non weight bearing measurement? Answer: 691

To tie this into Chapter 3 and 4 on gait and biomechanical examination, with achilles tendon problems, the most important examinations to do in 10 minutes (or 20 minutes) are:

- AJDF examination
- Single heel raises
- Functional hallux limitus
- Varus or Valgus torque seen in Gait or RCSP
- Hamstring Flexibility examination
- Limb Length Discrepancy (if picked up in Gait Evaluation)

Common Mechanical Changes for Achilles Tendon Injuries (with the common ones used in RED)

1. Cam Walker
2. Stretching for both gastrocnemius and soleus
3. Strengthening for both gastrocnemius and soleus
4. Heel lifts to take some pressure off the tendon
5. Athletic shoes with heel elevation if possible
6. Avoid negative heel positioning and stretching (where the heel is lower than the front of the foot)
7. Correction of varus or valgus heel positioning if present
8. Taping to support the Achilles
9. Rigid AFO

Cam Walker, and even full permanent casts, with crutches can be used in the acute phase for any degree of achilles tear or inflammation. Its mechanical function is purely in resting the injured tissue as much as possible. The exact diagnosis can take weeks, and may even require an MRI needing authorization. We want to drive the patient's pain to 0-2 as quickly as possible, and in doing so in the face of diagnosis still looming, we are protecting the patient. You are creating an environment for healing even when you plan on surgery or regenerative techniques now available.

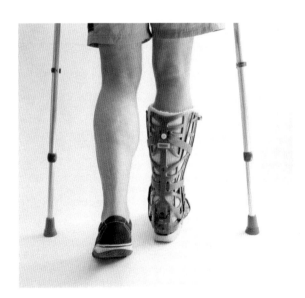

Stretching for both gastrocnemius and soleus is crucial when the achilles is tight, and a disservice to the patient when the achilles are normal length to over-flexible, or in the presence of a tear even unknown at the present time. Its mechanical function is to keep the tendon loose when the presence of pain tends to over tighten the tissue. You stretch the gastrocnemius with the knee fairly straight and the soleus with the knee bent over 20-25 degrees or more. Follow all the rules of stretching to be discussed in Chapter 11 of this Book 3. In general, avoid negative stretching (heel lower than the front of your foot) and painful stretching as you may be preventing the healing process of microtears.

Practical Biomechanics Question #351: Explain why in the case of an undiagnosed micro tear in the achilles tendon, why continuing to keep the pain level 5-7 is not an ideal protocol? Answer: 691

Strengthening for both gastrocnemius and soleus is really at the heart of lower extremity biomechanics due to the vital function of the achilles tendon. Its mechanical functions are to maintain posterior ankle stability and to enable a powerful gait and athletic functioning. My goal standard in achilles rehabilitation, but in most of my injuries, is to get the patient to do 25 one-sided straight knee heel raises (gastrocnemius), and 12 one-sided bent knee heel raises (soleus). Chapter 11 of this Book 3 will delve into this important exercise more thoroughly.

Practical Biomechanics Question #352: There is debate on whether the single leg balancing or heel raise is the most important exercise every patient should be doing. How much do you have to bend the knee to begin placing the stress on the soleus and off the gastrocnemius muscles? Answer: 691

Heel lifts to take some pressure off the tendon of normally ¼ inch due several positive mechanical changes. Its mechanical function is to both relax the achilles in standing and pre-load the tendon for better functioning in activities. Of course, this applies to heeled shoes also. First of all, they shorten the tendon making it easier to contract or activate, and secondly, they can shift the body weight slightly forward reducing the load on the tendon.

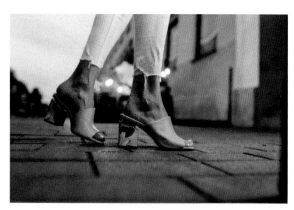

A very stable wider Cuban Heel definitely helps people walk more powerfully

Athletic shoes with heel elevation if possible are now considered the traditional shoes for running with 12-15 mm of heel height. Its mechanical function is the same as heel lifts just mentioned. This is about a ½ inch heel raise and really helps the achilles work well. The flatter the shoe, from zero drop to 4 mm, like the minimalist shoes, or the Altra or Hoka One One, take some pressure off the knees and ball of the foot but add load to the achilles. This is the opposite of what you typically want to do in the early treatment days of an achilles injury.

Practical Biomechanics Question #353: When you think mechanics, you should think in terms of how your mechanical changes affect the lower extremity in both positive and negative ways. Explain why a heel lift placed in a shoe puts increased stress on the plantar fascia, but this is minimized by a heeled shoe. Answer: 691

Avoid negative heel positioning and stretching (where the heel is lower than the front of the foot) is one of the fundamentals I use in treating achilles tendons. Its negative mechanical functions are that it crowds the tissue between the achilles and calcaneus, and over stretches both the healing tendon and sciatic nerve branches in the area. A negative achilles stretch is considered by some to produce a greater eccentric workout, and that may be so unless you are injured. As the heel drops down below the forefoot, the lower aspect of the achilles collides into the posterior superior aspect of the calcaneus. This loading does not happen in normal activities, and the compression force can lead to tendon and bursae issues. It also puts the achilles in a maximally stretched out vulnerable weakened position, and typically from this position is asked to contract strongly. Injury occurs if done repeatedly. This concept is especially true in insertional achilles tendonitis injuries with or without bone spurs.

VALGUS and VARUS deformity of the foot

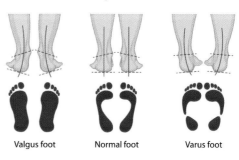

Valgus foot   Normal foot   Varus foot

The More Tilted the Heel, The More Stress on the Achilles Tendon to Function Properly

Correction of varus or valgus heel positioning if present lies behind the early work of Dr. Steven Subotnick, the "Running Foot Doc" who I first heard discuss this. The mechanical disadvantage of tilted heels is simply that the achilles will function twisted. The principle is that the achilles tendon is primarily a sagittal plane mover. If the foot is pronated too far from neutral subtalar joint, or if the foot is supinated from the neutral subtalar joint position, the achilles is torqued from the sagittal plane. Thus, the achilles has to function slightly twisted and strains easier.

Practical Biomechanics Question #354:The TC Angle between the tibia and calcaneus is also called the Achilles Angle. O degrees is where the tendon and heel line up perfectly. It is not uncommon to run with an Achilles Angle of +20 degrees (very pronated). Treatment therefore should be directed towards more varus positioning. What are 3 common methods of improving this varus positioning? Answer: 691

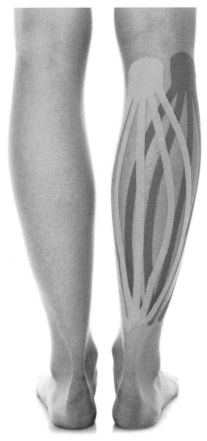

Here Achilles Tendon Taping is meant to be supportive to the tendon, but not restrictive

Taping to support the Achilles has many examples, but all in an attempt to slightly immobilize, or slightly support and take the strain off the tendon. Its mechanical function is to lessen the stress on the achilles, but maintain power and posterior ankle stability. My ideal taping is with a leukotape that starts under the heel, runs up the back of the heel, and splits going up the leg to mid calf or higher. You place the tape onto the foot with the ankle slightly plantar flexed. Leukotape needs an under tape called Coverall to protect the skin. It can be technically challenging so I show my patients the process with one of the stretchable tapes like RockTape, Kinesiotape, or KT tape. All these tapes go high up the calf to spread the force over a big area for more comfort as this will decrease pressure in any given location (Pressure = Force times Surface Area).

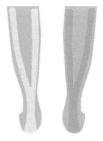

ACHILLES
KINESIOLOGY TAPING

Rigid AFO is normally seen in chronic situations where immobilization of the tendon is needed for a prolonged time. Its mechanical function is to rest the injured area while enabling function. In the case of achilles injuries, where possible operations are being put off for some reason, AFOs can allow some pretty normal activities and still protect the tendon.

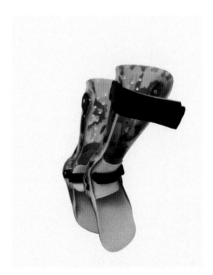

Here a Version of an AFO (Ankle Foot Orthosis)

Calf Strain

Calf Strain can be dramatic like pulling or pop of the medial head of the gastrocnemius (aka "Tennis Leg") to mild strain from overuse. The calf is comprised mainly of the more superficial and bigger gastrocnemius muscle bellies, and the smaller and deeper and lower soleus muscle bellies. The treatment of the calf can be the same as the achilles and typically simpler, with some fine tuning related to whether the gastrocnemius or the soleus is involved. Since the gastrocnemius crosses the knee, and can get pulled on with knee extension and hyperextension, training techniques may have to be tailored to a more flexed knee with a gastrocnemius tear, like lowering the seat of a cross training bicycle. Calf pain that is sudden, related to some sort of overuse, without a solid physical examination marked with common findings of a pulled muscle, should alert you to a possible posterior tibial stress fracture and the need for xrays. Sciatica, or some form of low back radiculopathy, can mimic calf strain but produced by neural tension.

To tie this into Chapter 3 and 4 on gait and biomechanical examination, with calf pain, the most important examinations to do in 10 minutes (or 20 minutes) are:

- Homan's test for DVT
- Straight Leg Testing for nerve involvement
- Observation of swelling or ecchymosis
- AJDF measurement
- Single Heel Raise Testing
- Signs of over pronation or over supination which produce varus and valgus torques.
- Tibial Compression Test for tibial stress fracture

Practical Biomechanics Question #355: Review the definition of the 3 Grades of Calf Strain. Answer: 691

Common Mechanical Changes for Calf Strain (with the common ones used in RED)

1. Cam Walkers with or without Crutches
2. Stretching of the gastrocnemius and soleus
3. Strengthening of the gastrocnemius and soleus
4. Calf mobilization therapy
5. Heel lifts to take some pressure off the tendons
6. Avoid negative heel positioning and stretching
7. Correction for varus or valgus positioning when abnormal
8. Taping to support the Achilles/calf

Cam Walkers with or without Crutches are used for the initial phase of rehabilitation to rest or immobilize the calf if the injury seems more severe than an overuse Grade 1 Strain. Grades 2 and 3 imply tearing of the tissue which will need time to repair without constant motion inhibiting that process. The mechanical function is to simply rest the injured tissues. Both the history of the acuteness and severity of disability, along with your physical examination, should help you decide if protection is necessary. Many times, 4 to 10 days of this type of immobilization helps the patient from re-tearing fibers, as the initial reparative process begins.

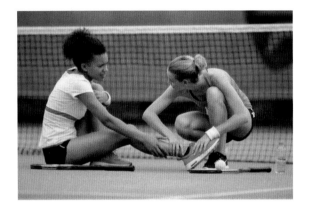

Stretching of the gastrocnemius and soleus is very crucial for calf injuries and right from the start of the injury in many minor injuries. The mechanical function is to prevent excessive tightness and scarring to occur which is common in the calf area. So many patients are afraid to pull the calf further with stretching, but if they can stretch and massage very easy with no pain it is so beneficial. The scarring post grade 2 calf strain greatly prolongs the healing if not stretched out. There should be no pain during or afterwards and it should be done 3-5 times daily. I find that most patients feel more comfortable leaving this decision to a physical therapist. The emphasis is on light stretching, not too long, not painful, and again shorter duration and multiple times times a day. You can stretch the muscles without weight bearing at first. The gastrocnemius is stretched the knee fairly straight, and the soleus is stretched with the knee bent over 20 degrees or greater.

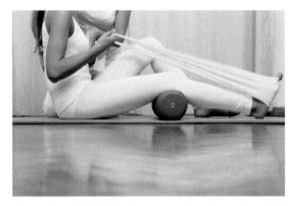

Here the Calf is being stretched gently with a Light Resistance band Non Weighting Bearing wrapped around the Foot

Practical Biomechanics Question #356: Injured muscles tighten up and this can be a cause of re-injury or just prolonged rehabilitation. Sports Medicine is built on a Foundation of early mobilization, including early strengthening and stretching of the tissues. What would be 4 keep points to emphasize to the athlete at your first encounter to begin safe stretching? A:691

Strengthening of the gastrocnemius and soleus is crucial as long as we can maintain good flexibility. Its mechanical function is to restore strength to the injured tissue as soon as possible. This is why being able to measure ankle joint dorsiflexion accurately is vital. Both an over flexible gastrocnemius or soleus, or an overly tight gastrocnemius or soleus, cause an inherent weakness of the tendon. It is so important to understand the force length curve of tendons and apply that to the achilles tendon. Both a tight achilles and an over stretched achilles have relatively poor strength or force it can generate. In a normal lower extremity rehabilitation program, 25 single heel raises with the knee straight (gastrocnemius) and 12 single heel raises with the knee bent (soleus) are the gold standards of good achilles strength. However, to get to this gold standard, you may have to work through all the levels of strengthening from muscle stimulation, active range of motion, isometric, progressive resistance, isotonic, and functional. Chapter 11 will explore this in greater detail.

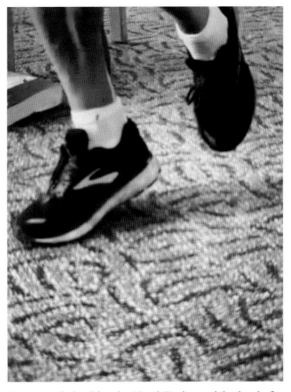

Here a right Single Heel Raise with the left foot off weighted. This is done knee straight for gastrocnemius and knee bent for soleus muscle fibers

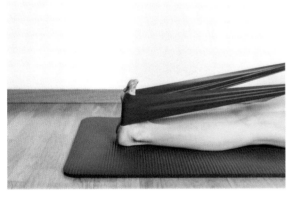

Resistance Band is used to strengthen the Gastrocnemius typically progressions from 2 sets of 10 reps slowly to 2 sets of 25 before moving to the next level of resistance

Calf mobilization therapy is vital in many cases of calf strain and chronic achilles issues. Its mechanical function is to break down excessive scar tissue and mobilize muscle knots and fluid accumulations. Yet, what is its primary purpose? Is it the breaking down of scar tissue? Is it the relaxation of muscle tension? Whatever is happening, several sessions of good calf mobilization work from a physical therapist or sports massage therapist can reduce pain in the calf and/or achilles for months at a time. I always love when they tell me what they found that was not right.

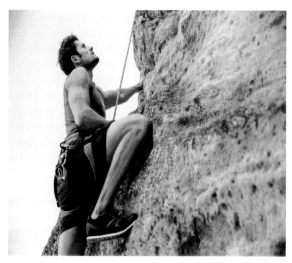

Heel lifts to take some pressure off the tendons definitely have been shown to reduce the load on the achilles and thus the calf. Their mechanical function is to decrease the stress to the calf, unless they cause too much knee flexion. And, unless you are treating a short leg, any heel lift on one side should be balanced by the other side. I will typically use ¼ inch lifts.

Practical Biomechanics Question #357: Many deep calf strains are caused by soleal weakness with over flexibility. Match that up with over knee flexion in a runner with tight hamstrings. Why do tight hamstrings cause us to use our soleus muscle much more than the stronger gastrocnemius?692

Avoidance of negative heel positioning and stretching is to be honored for several months with calf strain symptoms. The mechanical disadvantage of negative heel positioning is that you ask the tendon to contract from a weaker over stretched position. This is where you put the heel off a curb or stair lower than the front of the foot. But in activity, like walking up hills, you can get into this position easily and it should be minimized.

The patient has to analyze the positions that they get into to try to avoid this negative heel position for awhile

Correction for varus or valgus positioning when abnormal can be very helpful. The mechanical disadvantage of these frontal plane abnormal positions is that the tendon is functioning in a twisted position. I explain to my patients that the achilles/calf is a sagittal plane mover. It is designed to go forward. If you add frontal, and even transverse, plane tilts, the tissue has to work twisted and strain occurs.

Taping to support the Achilles/calf is a vital part of mechanical treatment and very successful. Its mechanical function is to support the calf muscle, and immobilize it slightly. This has been previously discussed with the achilles tendon.

Practical Biomechanics Question #358: If tight achilles/calf muscles are a cause of injury, why do we use heel lifts in their treatment which also can tighten the tissues? Answer: 692

Shin Splints

I love shin splints for the academic challenge to figure out what is wrong and what muscle/tendon, and sometimes bone, is involved. I breakdown shin splints into medial, lateral, anterior, and posterior. The muscles and tendons involved are summarized below for each.

Medial Shin Splints

Involves the posterior tibial tendon, flexor hallucis longus tendon, or the flexor digitorum longus tendon (and the soleus muscle attachment).

Lateral Shin Splints

Involves the peroneus longus tendon or the peroneus brevis tendon.

Anterior Shin Splints

Involves the anterior tibial muscle, extensor hallucis longus tendon, extensor digitorum longus tendon, or the peroneus tertius tendon.

Posterior Shin Splints

Involves the gastrocnemius muscle or the soleus muscle

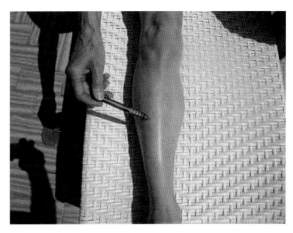

Common Location Anterior Shin Splints

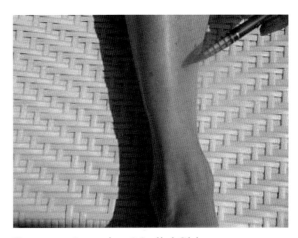

Common Location Medial Shin Splints

Practical Biomechanics Question #359: What is Occam's Law about treatment for shin splints? Answer: 692

Shin splints actually can be defined as pain between the ankle and the knee. There are alot of structures that can be involved which are important when treating these symptoms. When we treat shin splints, we can simply use activity modification, some ice, general leg strengthening, cross training, and most patients will do fine. For the patient who does not respond to simple measures, they could have compartment syndrome or tibial/fibular stress fractures. Muscle testing sometimes helps, but most cases of shin splints are related to a relatively normal muscle which fatigues when overused. It is hard to test in the office when the patient is rested for any muscle weaknesses, although you can have patients workout hard, or workout to the threshold of pain, before their appointment at the recommended end of the day. Chapter 11 will go over muscle testing principles, and one of them is to test the muscle in two basic positions: patient has advantage and examiner has advantage. You can pick up subtle weaknesses this way.

Practical Biomechanics Question #360: Which of the following is false regarding muscle testing. Answer: 692

1. Always test muscle strength early in the day
2. Always compare both the right and left sides
3. Examine a muscle both where the examiner has the advantage and the patient has the advantage
4. Test muscle strength even when there is severe pain

A thorough understanding of shin splints starts with you defining it as one of these 4 types. If the patient presents with medial tibial shin splints, the muscles involved are posterior tibial, flexor digitorum longus, flexor hallucis longus, and the soleus insertion. We then have to look for overuse in one of its functions. So, what do these muscles actually do? Since they all arise from the deep posterior compartment (not counting the soleal attachment), they are

ankle plantar flexors and ankle invertors. What is the primary ankle plantar flexor? That is the achilles tendon, but anything that makes the achilles tendon weak can cause you to overuse one of the 3 muscles causing medial shin splints. Typical weakness in the achilles is simply fatigue from the new sport they are engaging in, or just adding hills to their running program can fatigue the achilles. But, an over stretched achilles or excessive tight achilles, is considered weak by force length physics. With the recent craze of zero drop shoes, I have also seen more achilles and anterior or medial shin splints.

The inverter function is probably the more common cause of medial shin splints. What taxes the inversion strength of these muscles? Excessive Pronation can cause these 3 muscles to fatigue and strain as they attempt to decelerate the pronation, along with the achilles complex of gastrocnemius and soleus. As the arch collapses in pronation, the medial 3 are strained, but especially the posterior tibial and peroneus longus (a cause of lateral shin splints).

One of the causes of severe foot pronation is achilles tightness called equinus. This tightness can be the cause of posterior shin splints, but also anterior and medial shin splints. This is why a complete understanding of achilles strength and flexibility is crucial. If the achilles is tight, it is harder for the anterior (extensors) to dorsiflex the foot (thus causing anterior shin splints). If the achilles is tight, the foot can pronate and the arch collapses, both putting strain on the functions of the deep posterior compartment. If the achilles is tight, the forefoot is forcibly loaded by ground reactive force, making it difficult to bend the toes in propulsion. Stress is placed on the long flexors (medial shin splints) and long extensors (anterior shin splints).

One of the number one causes of shin splint type pain is undiagnosed stress fractures. The young inexperienced cross country runners who do not respond to shin splint treatment should be worked up for tibial (anterior or medial shin splints) stress fractures or fibular (lateral shin splints) stress fractures. This is still a version of the same process of overload. The overload in shin splints goes to the weakest link in the chain: the bone and a fracture occurs, the periosteum of the bone, the muscle belly, or the tendon. The five most common types of stress fractures which are mistaken for shin splints are: posterior tibial (posterior or medial shin splints), distal tibia (medial shin splints), anterior tibial (anterior shin splints), fibula (lateral shin splints), or proximal tibial (either medial or anterior shin splints). Of course, if you do make the diagnosis a stress fracture, always think about the overall bone health. Did this bone break not only due to the mechanical overload of hills, pronation, supination, tight muscles, etc, but is the bone actually healthy? An unhealthy bone becomes the weak link in the chain. A Vitamin D blood level is the first place to start.

The game for me is trying to figure out what muscle group is involved and what could be the cause of the overuse of that muscle/tendon. If we take the extensors as a group, they give us anterior shin splints. What causes general overload of the extensor group? The extensor group is again overloaded with a very tight achilles tendon complex which makes it work harder to flex the ankle joint. Also running hills makes you use the extensors differently than what you are used to, especially eccentrically as you run downhills as they avoid foot slap. Typically our bodies will get used to the activity, so shin splints are usually from new activities or changes in some routine. When shin splints occur in a seasoned runner for example, I think bone over tendon, therefore I want to rule out a stress fracture first. And, to add an extra twist, there are 4 individual extensor tendons. The anterior tibial tendon can cause a shin splint particularly if the foot pronates too much. The anterior tibial is straining to decelerate contact phase pronation. The peroneus tertius and extensor digitorum longus get painful with over supination especially in midstance or propulsion. While the extensor hallucis longus is fairly neutral to the subtalar joint, it can overload in functional hallux limitus as it tries to lift the big toe off the ground, or in painful big toe joints as protection.

The lateral shin splint syndrome is commonly caused by over firing of the peroneals to protect the lateral ankle. Common causes of normal lateral or foot overload are: laterally worn shoes, running on banked road (foot held supinated), shoes laterally unstable (70% of all supination problems are not in supinators structurally), and foot types like pes cavus that overly supinate. One of the exceptions to this concerns the function of peroneus longus tendon to raise the medial arch by plantar flexing the first metatarsal. Here lateral shin splints can develop from over pronation when the peroneus longus is strained.

The posterior shin splint is typically the soleus fibers or a tibial stress fracture. The pain is deep to the calf muscle belly, so given the name shin splint since it does not seem to be a calf strain. The stress fracture may never show up on x-ray, and not seem serious enough to get a conclusive MRI or Tc99 bone scan. Posterior Shin Splints involve understanding overload situations of the soleus primarily. The soleus plantar flexes the ankle, supinates the subtalar joint, and stabilizes the posterior aspect of the ankle. Posterior shin splints then involve attempts to plantar flex the ankle excessively (like excessive jumping jacks), or from abnormal positions (like those created by the introduction of hills), or during tremendous overload (like the early routines in ballet en pointe for a new season), or from a weak soleus.

Practical Biomechanics Question #361: Match the potential overload with the various shin splints listed. Answer: 692
- Lateral Shin Splint
- Medial Shin Splint
- Anterior Shin Splint
- Posterior Shin Splint
1. Excessive supination due to pes cavus
2. Excessive strain due to a weak achilles
3. Excessive pronation in pes planus
4. Excessive downhill running

To tie this into Chapter 3 and 4 on gait and biomechanical examination, with shin splints, the most important examinations to do in 10 minutes (or 20 minutes) are:
- Evaluation of Tendencies to Pronate or Supinate
- Ankle Joint Dorsiflexion for Equinus
- Evaluation of the Involved Muscle Group Strength
- When Long Flexors or Extensors Involved, look at the factors increasing Digital Instability like Forefoot to Rearfoot Alignment, Pes Cavus, Midtarsal Joint Looseness

Common Mechanical Changes for Shin Splints (with the common ones used in RED)
1. Strengthening of Involved Muscle Group
2. Stretching of the Involved Muscle Group
3. Reducing the Suspected Pronation or Supination Tendencies
4. Stretching the Achilles Complex
5. Strengthening the Achilles Complex
6. Custom Orthotic Devices particularly for Forefoot to Rearfoot Alignment Issues Involved
7. Training Decisions
8. Consideration of Bone Involvement

Strengthening of Involved Muscle Group is crucial in all 4 types of Shin Splints. Its mechanical function is to strengthen the muscles to take the load off the bone or to reduce some undesired motion. Chapter 11 will go over the muscle testing principles and you will need to learn how to differentiate the muscles in each group. This is typically well taught in Podiatry schools how to differentiate testing of the gastrocnemius and soleus in the posterior group, and the other muscle groups equally challenging. It is important to know if it is the posterior tibial, flexor hallucis longus, or flexor digitorum longus giving the medial ankle pain. Or, if it is the peroneus longus or brevis that hurts when testing against resistance. Or, if it is the anterior tibial or another one of the extensors producing the anterior shin splint. Every Podiatrist should understand the nuisances of individually testing the 11 muscle tendons around the ankle. There are 4 basic motions: dorsiflexion, plantarflexion, inversion, and eversion. Each one of these motions can be done in various positions to individually test muscles.

Practical Biomechanics Question #362: What motion of the ankle tests for the peroneus longus tendon? What motion of the ankle tests for the posterior tibial tendon? What motion of the ankle tests soleus over the gastrocnemius tendons? 692

Of course, after testing, we have to determine what level of strengthening program to prescribe. I will leave that task to Chapter 11.

Stretching of the Involved Muscle Group is typically only done for the anterior or posterior muscle/tendon groups, along you could include myofascial release treatment for the medial compartment and deep muscle massage to the lateral compartment. Its mechanical function is to relax tension in the involved muscles and their tendons.. Chapter 11 of this Book 3 will have the general rules for stretching, but remember stretching should never hurt or the tightness actually gets worse. I recommend stretching an involved group 3 times a day so I can get to 100 stretches within a month.

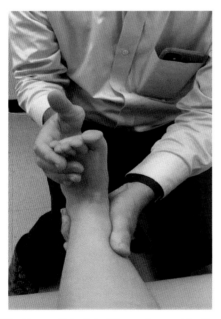

Testing of Ankle Eversion with the Ankle sagittal plane neutral while tell you the Peroneus Longus Strength

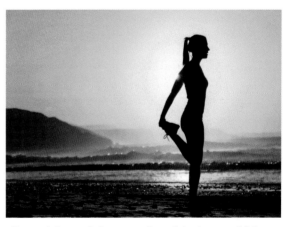

Stretching of the anterior shin by grabbing the toes and plantar flexing the ankle

Practical Biomechanics Question #363: We stretch to warm up tissue, attempt to reduce overly chronically tight tissue, and relax a sore area. Why would a muscle get tight when it is being overworked, like the anterior muscle group with too much downhill running? Answer: 692

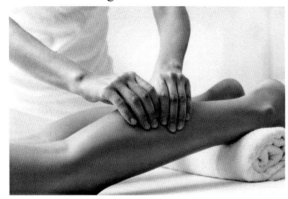

Deep Massage to stretch and relax the peroneal tendons when sore

Reducing the Suspected Pronation or Supination Tendencies with varus or valgus wedges, taping, arch supports, shoe changes, custom orthotics, and strengthening exercises occurs when you think the pronation or supination observed in gait or activity is related to the type of shin splint. Their mechanical function is to help tendons work less that are trying to help decelerate an undesired motion. This may be over pronation with fatigue and strain of the posterior tibial or anterior tibial tendons, or over supination with fatigue and strain of the peroneus longus and brevis tendons. The biomechanics of tendon injury is fascinating, and any help you can give to them will both speed recovery and decrease recurrence.

Practical Biomechanics Question #364: On a steep downhill, a hiker will start hurting at their weakest link. What is being strained in the act of going downhill when there's too little fat pad under the metatarsal heads?692

Stretching the Achilles Complex is vital to most sports injuries when there are equinus forces. Its mechanical function is to strengthen the muscle by making sure it is in the normal range of flexibility. A muscle too tight or too flexible is weak in functioning. However, it is so important to be able to reliably measure for this equinus because over stretching a normal or hyper flexible achilles tendon will do more harm than good. This concept has been fully explained in Chapter 4 of both Book 1 and Book 2. Tight achilles have been known to be involved in all 4 shin splint types.

Strengthening the Achilles Complex is vital when the achilles is weak. Its mechanical function is to make sure the achilles acts as the most powerful muscle/tendon in the body that it is to stabilize the ankle. The acid test for normal achilles strength is 25 single leg heel raises with the knee straight (gastrocnemius) and 12 single leg heel raises with the knee bent (soleus). These are typically done in the evening after the main activities of the day are over. The stronger we make the ankle, the more stress it can take in athletic activities.

Custom Orthotic Devices particularly for Forefoot to Rearfoot Alignment Issues Involved is your classic Root design. Its mechanical functions are to give the achilles tendon a very stable platform to push off from, and to prevent the pronation (medial or anterior shin splints) of forefoot varus feet and the supination (lateral shin splints) of forefoot valgus feet. Doctors not trained in Root biomechanics tend to use more metatarsal pads and anterior orthotic bars and posts, and combinations of all may be needed. Not only is forefoot support great for the correction of pronation or supination tendencies, the metatarsal support provided can be crucial for long flexor or extensor produced medial or anterior shin splints.

Training Decisions for shin splints is universally to lighten the load on the injured tissue. The mechanical function of various training decisions is to decrease some stresses through the foot and ankle. And for those athletes who seek treatment, the chance of an undiagnosed stress fracture is high due to the higher level of pain experienced in a stress fracture vs normal shin splints. The runner must cross train with biking as the mainstay alternative. Since both hill work and speed work is the most stressful, slow distance training is the first goal to accomplish. Each sport involved will have different strategies at lightening the stress first, and then gradually re-introducing these same stresses.

Practical Biomechanics Question #365: One of the best recommendations with patients with shin splints is to slow down or rest and cross train for a short time? If you think the medial shin splints are related to FDL overuse, what OTC device is helpful? 692

Consideration of Bone Involvement is very very important in shin splints. There are yearly reported cases of compound fractures in runners ignoring the shin splint symptoms only to have the stress fracture become a through and through fracture. I

have had 27 year olds with shin splints have the bone density of 80 year olds. It is important to remember Shin Splints can be bone pain primarily, and verifying the patient has good bone health is crucial.

Practical Biomechanics Question #366: Any case of medial, lateral, or anterior shin splints that is not improving in one month time should have what test (besides x-rays) to look at bone health? Answer: 693

Tibial Stress Fractures

One of the first points I would like to make is that tibial stress fractures are normally caused by overuse and certain motions more than excessive impact. In Book 1, I discussed the concept of Rule of 3, highlighting that most injuries have 3 or more causes that collide into a "perfect storm" causing an injury. Of these 3 or more causes, one may be far the most important to the causation of the injury. Possible causes of tibial stress fractures therefore can be impact shock in an overuse pattern, over pronation tendencies, over supination tendencies, overall bone health issues, and excessive forward bend.

There are 4 common areas on the tibia where you can develop tibial stress fractures and each with a different biomechanics which are related to overuse. The 4 areas are: distal medial tibia just above the medial malleolus, the posterior border often misdiagnosed as calf pain, the proximal medial area where the tibial shaft is becoming the medial tibial plafond, and the anterior crest. The 5th common tibial stress fracture occurs at the tibial and medial malleolus junction typically related to an inversion ankle sprain so more acute in nature.

The distal medial tibial stress fractures tend to be from some combination of impact and excessive supination where the medial side of the ankle is bearing more weight. Here the medial side of the talus and the tibia meet with contact phase subtalar joint supination. The prolonged excessive talar inversion on the tibial causes the development of overuse bone reactions or stress risers. This is the same basic mechanism on an acute inversion ankle sprain leading to medial malleolar stress fracture or full frank fractures.

The posterior tibial stress fractures tend to be from excessive pronatory torque and muscle contractions to decelerate that motion. Over pronation is the most common cause with the posterior tibial muscle fibers or the soleus muscle fibers pulling so hard to decelerate the pronation that stress fractures can occur. When the bone does not break, but the same muscle pull causes a larger area of bone to get inflamed, it is called Medial Tibial Stress Syndrome (MTSS).

The proximal medial tibial stress fractures impact and excessive supination where the tibia and medial femoral condyles collide repeatedly. And, of course, it is the weakest link in the chain that gets injured, as the same motion can beat up the medial knee compartment.

The anterior crest tibial stress fractures are from straight impact where the tibia bows anteriorly and stress fractures can occur. I saw a professional ballet dancer (male) who had chronic shin pain from a recent tour in Europe. When x-rayed, he had several stress fractures that were new and several that were old and healed on each leg. It turns out that the stages in Europe are more raked, or slanted forward, than in the US, so the dancer had more bowing of the tibia each time he landed on the stage, often with the weight of a ballerina added that he was lifting.

Practical Biomechanics Question #367: What are the 4 common overuse tibial stress fracture locations, and which one is commonly related to over pronation? A:693

To tie this into Chapter 3 and 4 on gait and biomechanical examination, with tibial stress fractures, the most important examinations to do in 10 minutes (or 20 minutes) are:

- Signs of Excessive Pronatory Torque
- Signs of Poor Shock Absorption
- Signs of Excessive Supination
- Overall Subtalar Joint Motion
- RCSP
- Midtarsal Joint Motion

Practical Biomechanics Question #368: Why would subtalar joint motion be implicated in tibial stress fractures? Why would an inverted heel in RCSP possibly cause a tibial stress fracture? A: 693

Common Mechanical Changes for Tibial Stress Fractures (with the common ones used in RED)

1. Simple to Complex Pronatory Measures
2. Simple to Complex Supinatory Measures
3. Pure Shock Absorption Inserts
4. Shock Absorption Shoe Recommendations
5. Heel Cushions
6. Leg Strengthening Exercises
7. Support Hose/Compression Hose
8. Appropriate Stretching Exercises
9. Shoe Selection
10. Training Techniques
11. Limb Length Discrepancy Lifts for Short Leg

Simple to Complex Pronatory Measures have all been discussed in Chapter 5. Their mechanical function is to reduce the amount, velocity, or duration of abnormal motion that can stress the bone. I try to balance the varus support for pronation problems with cushion (to add some shock absorption). Therefore, if I make custom orthotic devices, the Hannafords for their shock absorption qualities would be my top choice. I can varus wedge with the Hannafords for pronation support all I want. The Hannafords are the king of shock absorption inserts.

Practical Biomechanics Question #369: All stress fractures have to be evaluated for torque and shock. Gait evaluation walking and/or running can typically help you decide what to do, but when the patient hurts, may have to be postponed. What are 3 biomechanical observations made just be having the patient stand in front of you that could indicate over pronation when running? Why should they bring in old worn down shoes for you to look at? A: 693

Simple to Complex Supinatory Measures are also discussed in Chapter 5. Their mechanical function is to reduce or eliminate the motion you believe is causing stress along the bone. When you supinate, you also rob the body of its natural shock absorption of normal subtalar joint pronation at contact with the group. So, the goal of this treatment is not to stop supination only, but to both stop supination and introduce pronation. This, of course, is best done with a custom device, but if we can stop supination and add some shock absorbing material, this is my second choice that can work.

The second common reason is that over supination at the subtalar and ankle areas causes the talus to collide with the medial aspect of the ankle joint (possibly overuse stress fracture), or that supination force jamming the medial tibial platfond into the femur. This will possibly cause proximal medial tibial stress fractures.

Practical Biomechanics Question #370: Why is some contact phase pronation good for shock absorption? .Answer: 693

Pure Shock Absorption Inserts only help slightly in my practice. Their mechanical function is to reduce impact stress on the foot and leg. I love Spenco, or one of its knockoffs (like ⅛ inch neolon), and poron is another good material. These materials work the least as a flat insert, as they only contact a small percentage of the body, and work the best attached to an arch support for better foot contact.

Shock Absorption Shoe Recommendations are exploding in the marketplace. Their mechanical function is to add impact shock absorption. It is so easy to have your athletes, even your severe pronators, rotating shoes to vary stresses. Most, if not all, of the tibial stress fractures are related to repetitive stress which you can vary with the same insert, but have them wear a variety of at least 2 shoe types. The maximalist shoes with their thick and soft midsole may be at the top, but shoes with both stability and cushion like the Brooks Ghost, New Balance 840, etc, are not far behind.

Heel Cushions and soft heel cups are one of the mainstays with tibial stress fractures. Their mechanical function is also for shock absorption at heel strike. When a patient comes in with a suspected tibial stress fracture, and gait shows poor shock absorption, starting the patient on some sort of simple heel cushion at the first visit can really help. If you are sure the problem is not a torque problem, consider also removing any hard post if they are orthotic wearers. The same would be to eliminate clunky heeled shoes which can add to ground reactive forces. The difference in heel stress can be much worse in heeled shoes than a wedge. Just remember, unless you are also treating a short leg problem, always put the heel cushion (or make a change in the heel area at all) on both sides for symmetry.

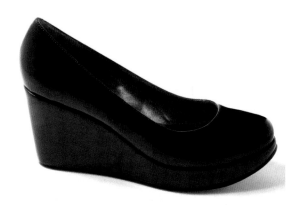

Wedged Shoes Distribute Stress Better than Heeled Shoes

Practical Biomechanics Question #371: Why in sports do heel cushions work less effectively than with standing activities?

Leg Strengthening Exercises greatly improve the stability of the skeletal structures around them, and absorb shock away from the bones. Their mechanical function is to take the stress away from the bones they surround. The muscles bulk up with exercise, even with simple active range of motion, and can protect the bones. Even though Re-Strengthening is Phase II of Rehabilitation, I love to start strengthening the muscle in the area (typically 4 directions at the ankle), and also strengthen the entire lower extremity as muscles distal and proximal to an injury can also be supportive and protective. Chapter 11 in this book will address strengthening exercises in more detail.

Practical Biomechanics Question #372: Are isotonic exercises more powerful than progressive resistive exercises? A: 693

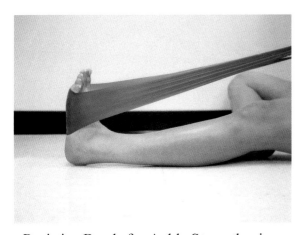

Resistive Bands for Ankle Strengthening

Support Hose/Compression Hose are being utilized in a different function than just venous return (which of course is also important). Their mechanical functions are in low level support to the tissues, and venous return to prevent stagnation of swelling. Support hose provides low grade support to the fascia and muscles for better function. Sports compression hose or socks (knee high) are very popular in the athletic world.

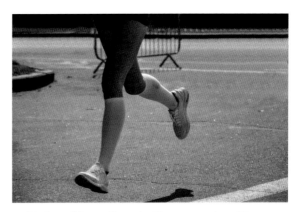

Below Knee Sports Compression Hose

Appropriate Stretching Exercises depend on what tibial stress fracture presents. Their mechanical function is to alleviate stress caused by tight muscles. If it is pronatory torque that causes a posterior tibial stress fracture with tight achilles added to the pronation, then calf stretches are crucial. If it is anterior tibial stress fractures from tight calf, or tight extensor compartments, your physical examination should tell you which, if not both, to stretch out.

Practical Biomechanics Question #373: Why would a tight achilles tendon cause the development of an anterior tibial stress fracture? Answer: 693

Shoe Selection will again depend on whether you decide that the problem is related to excessive pronatory torque (stability or motion control shoes), shock absorption (neutral or cushioned shoes), or both (maximalist shoes with stability). Their mechanical function depends on what function is needed. Shoes are a great help for us since they can do so many functions in their range of selection. The heel height can be varied along with the amount of cushion or the amount of varus support. It can be fun thinking of the aspects of a shoe that can help an individual athlete.

Training Techniques again will focus on pronatory torque, lateral instability, or poor shock absorption. Their mechanical function is to avoid too much of anything. As you listen to the routine training schedule of the athlete, you will have a portrait of excess shock (straight overuse on cement or asphalt) or excess torque (overuse of rotation like side to side court sports, running on a slanted beach, or always running with or against traffic) painted for you. You will then add straight overuse, like too many miles or workout hours. If you had the history of winter sports, or a history of low Vitamin D, the bone health component to injury may be suspect. Another common use of overuse is working out when you are fatigued, since fatigued muscles will not protect bones well. The list of these training flaws could fill a book, but sometimes just listening can point you in the right direction.

Practical Biomechanics Question #374: Why does habitually running against traffic cause pronatory problems on the right leg of runners? Answer: 693

Limb Length Discrepancy Lifts for Short Leg is typically used when the long leg is putting excess stress on that leg. Their mechanical function is to balance abnormal stresses from right to left. Gait evaluation typically shows limb dominance (or more pressure on that side). The tibia broke either from this increased pressure or at least is aggravated by this pressure. Also, the long leg with its more compression forces, may also have excessive torque as this side pronates to lower the overall hip height. This excessive pronatory torque may be the true reason the tibia broke in the first place.

Fibular Stress Fractures

Fibular stress fractures tend to be caused by the excessive supination in a repetitive motion. I use the classic example of a professional ballerina who broke her fibula three times in 3 different places before seeking my advice to describe this problem. She did have low Vitamin D at one point that had been reversed. I watched her walk and she had normal biomechanics (no tendency to supinate or pronate excessively). All of our athletes are told to bring in their workout shoes, so then I evaluated her barre routine in the treatment room. It was obvious that she sickled (over supination) en pointe in various releve positions. This was not common of course in a professional dancer, but she said she had been aware of this problem and had spent the last few years trying to correct this mechanical fault. What is common was that though the treatment of 3 fibular stress fractures that her treating physicians had not made this connection. One of the differences in having a biomechanics based practice is that you are always looking for the mechanical causes or aggravating factors to an injury. This dancer was treated with a thick thread sewn on the lateral corner of the tip of her pointe shoes and this corrected the sickling issue. She danced for 2 more years before going off to medical school without another fibular stress fracture.

To tie this into Chapter 3 and 4 on gait and biomechanical examination, with fibular stress fractures, the most important examinations to do in 10 minutes (or 20 minutes) are:

- Gait signs of Excessive Supination
- RCSP
- Forefoot to Rearfoot Deformities
- Peroneal Strength

Common Mechanical Changes for Fibular Stress Fractures (with the common ones used in RED)

1. Poor Bone Health questions on low Vitamin D or overall bone density (with testing if there are any concerns)
2. Orthotic Devices
3. OTC Inserts or Valgus Wedges
4. Training Errors Correction
5. Peroneal Strengthening
6. Taping
7. Ankle Bracing
8. Gait Training
9. Shoe Advice and Selection
10. Widen Base of Gait

Poor Bone Health questions on low Vitamin D or overall bone density (with testing if there are any concerns) is always important with bone injuries. Its mechanical function is to make sure that the skeletal structure is sound. I always ask myself if the stress fracture should occur from straight overuse, and if not, perhaps a bone itself is weak for some reason. The fibula, like any long bone, can develop weak spots in the curves: both convex and concave. The fibula on x-ray may show multiple bends and curves that set up the ideal situation in overuse for a stress fracture. But, getting Vitamin D or bone density tests may be appropriate and definitely a vital part of the overall body's mechanics.

Orthotic Devices are utilized all the time to stop the severe forces of supination especially during the contact phase. Their mechanical function is to make a supinator into a normal pronator. This contact phase supination is decelerated by the peroneal tendons that at times pull so hard that the bone breaks. The common components that make up an orthotic device for supinators include: any everted forefoot deformity corrections, high lateral heel cups, extended lateral heel post, lateral phalanges, Denton modifications, Feehery cuboid support, cuboid pads, forefoot valgus forefoot extensions, and setting the original correction everted 2-3 degrees. All these will be discussed in Chapter 13 of Book 4.

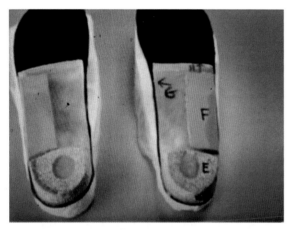

In designing orthotic devices for supination, what is "F"?

Practical Biomechanics Question #375: If we are designing an orthotic device to prevent excessive supination, why is a forefoot valgus deformity better to support than a forefoot varus deformity? A: 693

OTC Inserts or Valgus Wedges can be used to fight the excessive supination instability. Their mechanical function can be a simple method of eliminating excessive supination. The difference between a wedge and an OTC insert is that the insert may be better at overall foot stability and the wedge just for the frontal plane lateral instability. Both can help with this instability, thus both can improve pain produced by excessive peroneal tendon firing. The peroneus brevis stabilizes the lateral ankle and foot, and the peroneus longus stabilizes the lateral ankle, lateral rearfoot, cuboid, and medial arch. It can be complex enough that you have to eventually valgus wedge an arch support at times. You are customizing an OTC insert.

Training Error Correction means both to stop overuse techniques, but also to correct positions that place too much stress on the lateral ankle. Their mechanical function is typically to decrease the lateral ankle stress causing peroneal contractions. The more the lateral ankle is stressed, the stronger the peroneal tendons fire, the more possibilities of fibular stress fractures developing. This typically means decreasing the angle of cuts in sport drills, decreasing the time doing lateral work, and slowing down the side to side activities.

Practical Biomechanics Question #376: My first case of a patient with a fibular stress fracture on his right side. Was he habitually running with or against traffic? A: 693

Peroneal Strengthening means that the stronger the peroneal tendons are, the greater ability that they have to keep the stress off the bone. One of the primary mechanical functions is to take stress away from the bone it helps support. Normal muscle strength protects the underlying bone, unless the bone itself is weak. As the tendon weakens, the more it allows the ankle to be distorted, the more it has to overfire to attempt ankle protection. This overfiring can cause fibular stress fractures if the bone is the weak link in this scenario. Remember abnormal muscle firing, especially when weak and still trying to function, can cause abnormal stress on the muscle, tendon or bone. The area that complains first is the one that is the weakest link.

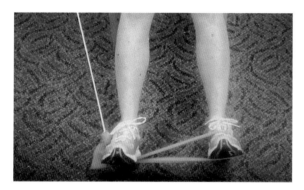

Resistance Band for Peroneal Strengthening

Taping for fibular stress fractures can be immobilization of the area with circumferential taping with some medial opening for swelling. Its mechanical functions are to either support the area that has broken, or prevent the inversion motion that increases peroneal muscle pull on the injury. The circumferential tape usually starts high medial, comes down across the fracture site, and goes back up medially as in a sling. This taping is normally with KT tape or RockTape. The more classic tape is to relax the pull of the peroneals on the fibula. It is called a J Strap and leukotape is utilized (the basic opposite of the Posterior Tibial Taping previously described).

Coverall is first utilized to cover the skin as leukotape can rip skin due to its strong pull. The tape is applied from under the medial malleolus, under the heel, and then up the lateral side of the leg normally ⅔ or more towards the knee. Then leukotape, which is slightly narrower than coverall, is applied gently over the skin from medial malleolus to lateral heel, and then a firmer pull all the way up the lateral side of the leg. Typically, the heel is slightly everted from its neutral position with the tibia while the leukotape is being pulled up the leg. This may stay on for 2-3 days at a time. This is a wonderful way to get good immobilization of inversion as activities anticipated will put higher demands on the lateral ankle.

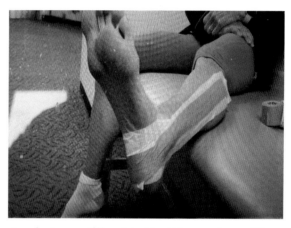

Leukotape utilized to limit inversion of the Ankle and Subtalar joints

Practical Biomechanics Question #377: Tape has also been known as "flexible casting" and can be very powerful at helping patients. I love to tape my athletes, and there is usually a way that can help any injury you face. In the photo of the leukotape above, where does the tape start medially? Answer: 694

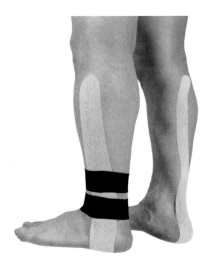

Here the left leg has KT tape for inversion support and black cross bands for injury support

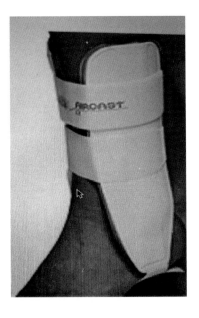

Aircast Stirrup Brace with air inflated medially and laterally

Ankle Bracing in general are pronators across the subtalar joint and immobilize the ankle joint. Their mechanical function is in some form of immobilization of the pull of the ankle muscles. There is a good probability that any of these will help fibula pain. However, I have long favored the original Aircast Stirrup brace and I put as much air as I can fit in the shoe for fibular stress fractures.

Practical Biomechanics Question #378: Explain how an ankle brace can take pressure off an injured area by limiting muscle contractions, compared to the principle of limiting motion in one area can create motion or stress in another area. 694

Gait Training is crucial when there are varus stresses to the gait walking and/or running that you want to be reduced. Its mechanical function is to reduce the lateral overload on the ankle and foot in both static and kinetic activities. Patients may have too narrow a base of gait which can be widened. Runners are notorious for a negative base of gait with high amounts of "running limb varus". Typically a skilled PT trained in gait analysis and corrections can help. However, there may be something the athlete does that puts too much lateral stress in workouts, like overstriding or lifting stance at the gym, that can be reduced.

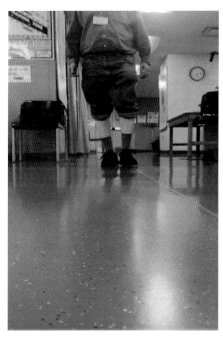

Watch Gait and Whether Cross Over Occurs Patient Here Moving Left Side Forward

Shoe Advice and Selection is also based on reducing varus stresses at the ankle and lower leg. The mechanical function is to minimize varus, while allowing all other normal motions to occur. Most agree that fibular stress fractures are produced by muscular tension, whereas tibial stress fractures are produced either by muscular tension or impact load. Classically, you want the patient in more neutral shoes, than stability shoes that may place varus stresses. As podiatrists, we are pretty skilled at deciding this, and it may take a patient bringing several shoes into the office to evaluate. Many pronators in years past were placed in motion control shoes and orthotics, only to become supinators with too much varus stresses. When you use orthotic devices, especially corrective ones, you do not want the shoe to do more than light stability and good shock absorption, unless you are dealing with severe pronation.

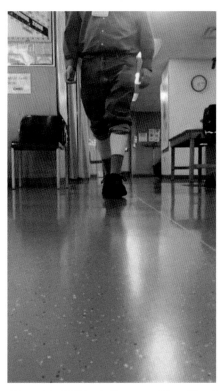

Here Left Heel Contact Too Far in Front of Right with Too Much Varus Alignment of Foot to Ground

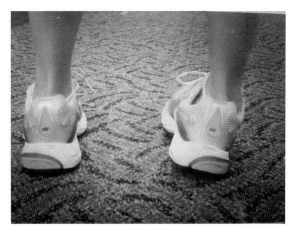

Here too soft a Shoe Laterally can produce Excessive Supination (seen on the right shoe)

Widen Base of Gait essentially places our body weight more medial on each foot, taking the strain off the fibula. Its mechanical function is to transfer weight and stress more medially. It is fairly easy to do this standing, like when cooking for long hours, but also in some of the gym workouts where it is okay (per your trainer) to widen your base squatting, weight lifting, etc. Sometimes this simple mechanical change can greatly speed up the rehabilitative process. I just talked about the same principle in Gait Training where the more narrow your base, the more stress on your fibula.

Practical Biomechanics Question #379: As you narrow your base of gait, the tibia gets more varus positioned to the ground, increasing the lateral stress on the ankle and leg. As you widen your base of gait, the tibia gets into a more valgus position to the ground, increasing the medial stresses on the ankle and lower leg. This is the same pattern with over supination and over pronation of the subtalar joint. Explain then how narrowing the base of gait is like excessive supination of the subtalar joint in its effect on lateral ankle stability. A: 694

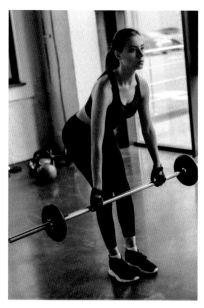

Here WeightLifter with Too Narrow Base overloading Laterally

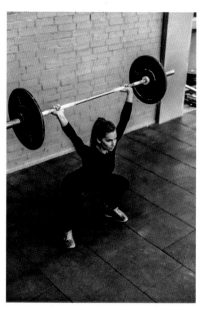

Appropriate Wide Base of Support for Even Weight Distribution Medially and Laterally

Patello-Femoral Pain Syndrome

The weaker vastus medialis allows the stronger vastus lateralis to pull the kneecap (patella) laterally subluxing it out of its groove. It is such a problem in most sports that it is called runner's knee, biker's knee, dancer's knee, etc. This tracking problem can start with foot pronation driving the knee medially and into some valgus giving the vastus lateralis the mechanical advantage over the smaller vastus medialis. Or, this tracking problem can start higher up with a weakness in the glutes and other external hip rotators that decelerate the internal motion of the femur attempting to keep it from going too far. There are braces and taping designed to prevent that subluxation laterally of the kneecap. Using orthotic devices with inversion built in can be a must for the running motion. Root balanced orthotic devices to vertical, with or without Kirby Skives, can help when the shoe is a motion control variety. 1/8th inch varus midsole wedges to a motion control shoe can be needed. Bike shops know how to varus wedge the cleat when motion analysis reveals that the knee moves too close to the bike frame (too internal). Ballet pointe shoes can need just a thicker thread sewn medially at the pointe of the shoe to prevent over pronation called "winging" while the dancer works on her technique and muscle strength. The world of sports medicine agrees to approach this problem from the hip, from the knee, and from the foot. All three areas can be essential.

To tie this into Chapter 3 and 4 on gait and biomechanical examination, with patello-femoral pain syndrome, the most important examinations to do in 10 minutes (or 20 minutes) are:

- Internal Knee Rotation in Gait and Static Examination
- Overall Quadriceps and Hamstring Strength, especially VMO
- Overall Quadriceps and Hamstring Flexibility
- External Hip Rotator Strength and Overall Hip Range of Motion
- Signs of Abnormal Pronation in Gait and Examination
- RCSP and NCSP

Common Mechanical Changes for Patellofemoral Pain Syndrome (with the common ones used in RED)

1. McConnell Taping
2. Patellar Bracing
3. Quadriceps strength especially short arc quads and single leg press (kneecap slightly turned out to emphasize vastus medialis)
4. Hamstring strength
5. Vastus lateralis stretching
6. Medial hamstring stretching
7. External Hip Rotator strengthening
8. Varus Wedges or Custom Orthotic Devices to help control excessive internal patellar rotation
9. Shoe Selection
10. Gait Training
11. Avoid Deep Knee Bend Positions

McConnell Taping was named after the originator, a PT from Australia, who introduced Leukotape and Coverall to pull the kneecap medially in activities. Its mechanical function is to put a medial moment on the knee cap preventing lateral subluxation. It has been one of the hallmarks of treatment for decades. Everyone should learn the classic McConnell Tape Technique.

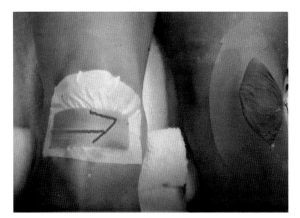

Classic McConnell Taping with Luekotape and Coverall

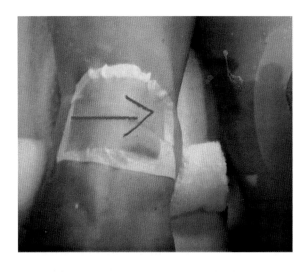

Typically 2 layers of Coverall are used to protect the skin and then 1-2 layers of Leukotape are anchored laterally and pulled medially

Practical Biomechanics Question # 380: The pain from PFD can be excruciating where McConnell taping is too uncomfortable. As the symptoms calm down, McConnell taping can be vital in the rehabilitative process. Explain why the patella naturally will subluxate laterally.

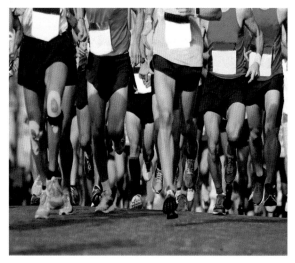

Presently I see more of the Kinesiotape Version Surrounding the Patella medially and laterally, and then a piece to Stablize the Patellar Base

Patellar Bracing will typically have a hole for the kneecap to sit in and prevent abnormal tracking. Its mechanical function is to give external support to the knee and help prevent motion of the patella is the transverse plane. The one I use is called Genutrain by Bauerfiend.

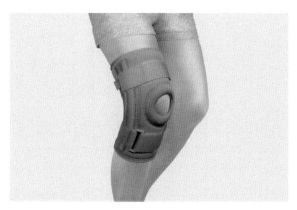

Patellar Stabilizing Brace

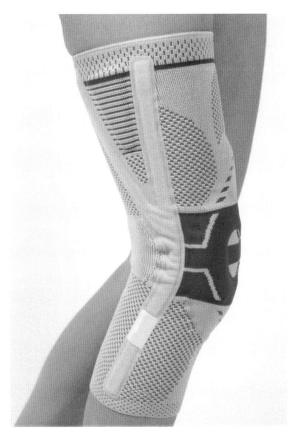

Bauerfiend Genutrain Brace

Practical Biomechanics Question #381: What is the main purpose of the two velcro straps in the knee brace above? A: 694

Quadriceps strength, especially short arc quads and single leg press (kneecap slightly turned out to emphasize vastus medialis) also one of the hallmarks of treatment. The mechanical function is to attempt to eliminate the huge muscle imbalance presence between the vastus medialis and the much stronger vastus lateralis. The weaker vastus medialis must be strengthened along with stretching of the vastus lateralis.

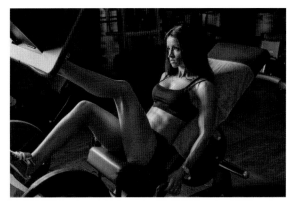

Single Leg Press is one of the most Powerful ways of Strengthening the Vastus Medialis but also Identifying its Strength

Hamstring strength is of course different then tightness. We need that 50% ratio of hamstring to quadriceps strength, and in this case, we need to focus on lateral hamstring strength slightly more than medial hamstring. The mechanical function of the hamstrings is to avoid hyper-extension of the knee which irritates the back of the kneecap. Hamstring curls are the primary exercise utilized.

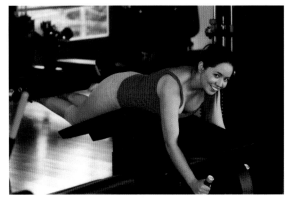

The use of Hamstring Curls to keep these muscles strong

Vastus lateralis stretching is so crucial as the lateral quadriceps, iliotibial band, and lateral fascia all are implicated in pulling the patella laterally and causing lateral subluxation symptoms. The mechanical function of the stretching is to relax the powerful lateral pull at the kneecap. It is extremely important to use the opposite hand to perform this stretch properly.

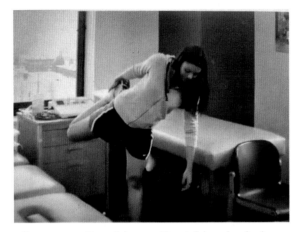

Improper Quadriceps Stretching includes unstable while occurring, using same hand and foot, and bending knee too much

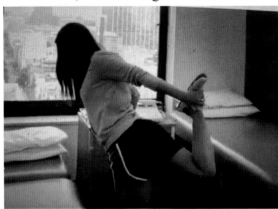

Proper Quadriceps Stretching includes holding on for stability, using opposite hand and foot, and never bending knee past 90 degrees

Medial hamstring stretching is important when excessively tight. A tight medial hamstring will internally rotate and flex the knee making it unstable. Remember that it is this internal knee rotation that can put the kneecap in a vulnerable position

whereas lateral subluxation can occur. The mechanical function of medial hamstring stretching then is to lessen the medial position of the kneecap.

Practical Biomechanics Question #382: What are 7 common general rules for stretching any muscle/tendon complex? 694

Practical Biomechanics Question #383: Is is tight medial or lateral hamstrings that increase internal knee rotation? A: 695

Practical Biomechanics Question #384: What are common causes of not being able to stretch out tight muscles? A: 695

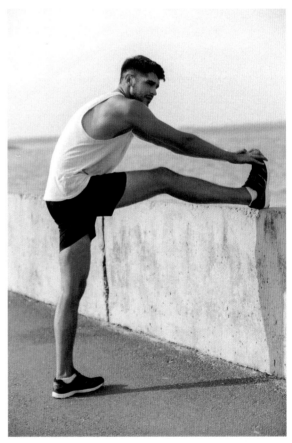

This runner is demonstrating the classic hamstring stretch. If you turn your foot inward while doing this stretch, you will stretch the medial hamstring more.

External Hip Rotator strengthening has been a 40 year battle of the Physical Therapy world who have felt it even more important than VMO strengthening for patello-femoral issues. There are so many great external hip rotators. These include: gluteus minimus and medius, iliopsoas, and piriformis. Strengthening these muscles help hold the knee more central, as it is the internal position and rotation that allows for the lateral subluxation to occur. The mechanical function of external hip rotator strengthening is to help position the knee cap in a more neutral position.

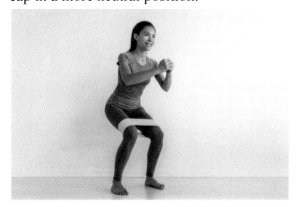

Classic External Hip Rotation Strengthener where the patient is asked to rotate their knees external. If they are internal naturally, they can center their knees and slide side to side maintaining that center position.

Varus Wedges or Custom Orthotic Devices to help control excessive internal patellar rotation has been another 40 year battle of Podiatrists and finally recognized as a vital part of the conservative treatment of knee pain. The key emphasis is in changing the foot position into more varus positioning to the ground. The mechanical function of custom orthotic devices or varus wedges is to help align the foot under the knee better (especially when the knee is too internal or the foot is too everted from subtalar neutral).

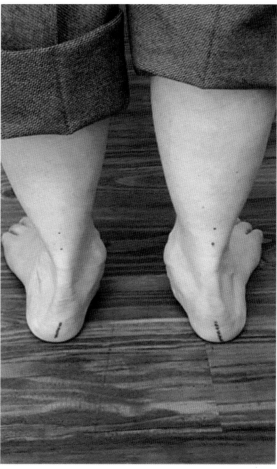

Here this very pronated patient with heel valgus or severe eversion needs varus re-aligning orthotic devices to help center the knee better. The same is true if the feet were not so bad, but the knee very internally rotated due to femoral anteversion.

Shoe Selection becomes crucial, and can not be separated from orthotic devices, to control excessive pronation and symptoms. The more support the shoe gives you, the less support is needed from the orthotic device, and vice versa.

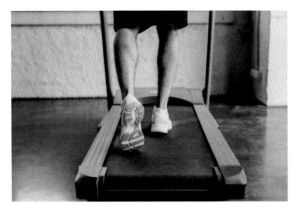

Shoes are a big part of Podiatry and our assessment and treatment. Many Podiatrists even have treadmills in their office for better visualization. The better the shoe is at achieving good stability, the less work the orthotic devices have to do.

Gait Training would be designed to decrease pronatory forces at the knee. Widening of the base of gait (not in genu valgum patients), shortening the stride, slowing the speed, are all typical components of gait training while the symptoms are rampant. The common use of hiking poles, when the knee is very sore, is a common way to redistribute the force.

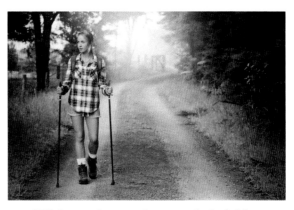

Hiking poles can be very helpful in redistributing weight in the early days of the Return to Activity Phase.

Avoid Deep Knee Bend Positions is related to the fact that over 40 degrees of knee bend, the pressure between the sore patella and femur increases every degree. Avoiding long sessions of this heightened knee internal pressure can help control symptoms. The secret is to keep everything short arc from +5 to +40-45 degrees.

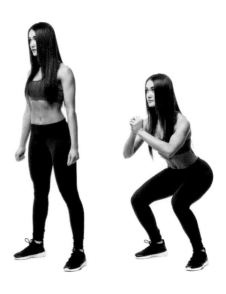

Here the athlete can attempt to control
the depth of her squat to accomplish
the short arc nature.

Practical Biomechanics Question #385:
Which of the following hip muscles does
not help patello-femoral tracking issues?

1. Adductor Longus
2. Piriformis
3. Gluteus Minimus
4. Iliopsoas
5. Sartorius A: 695

Medial Knee Compartment Syndrome

When I first started working at Saint Francis Memorial Hospital's Center For Sports Medicine, the only podiatrist in an orthopedic clinic, I spent almost 2 years only seeing knee problems. This is one of my favorite stories. The orthopedist, primarily Dr. James Garrick, had patients with medial knee joint line pain but were not locking, buckling, and could limit their pain. However, this was not without disability. I would watch him carefully evaluate the patient, place them on a PT strengthening program, and assign them to me for off weighting the medial compartment. One of the ironies was that podiatrists were taught the opposite of orthopedists in those days for this problem. I was taught that pronation causes closed kinetic chain tibial inversion with narrowing of the medial joint line, thus the treatment would be a varus wedge. Orthopedists were taught to pronate the patients with this problem, so utilized valgus wedges in an attempt to open up the medial joint line. What worked? Well, both worked 50% of the time alleviating symptoms, so when my varus wedge did not help I would turn the wedge over and make it a valgus wedge. Therefore, I was 100% successful in alleviating symptoms, some still needed surgery, and some have been coming back for 35 plus years for more wedges. Sadly, I saw this disappear with the modern orthopedist in my practice, who would simply get an MRI and schedule surgery. If you are over 40 years old, your MRI will show something to operate on most definitely..

To tie this into Chapter 3 and 4 on gait and biomechanical examination, with medial compartment knee symptoms, we are looking for signs of supination which can cause compression forces, or pronatory signs that make indicate excessive torque or compression forces, and the most important examinations to do in 10 minutes (or 20 minutes) are:

- Signs of Contact Phase Supination
- Forefoot to Rearfoot Deformities
- Metatarsal Alignment
- Peroneal Strength
- RCSP and NCSP
- Signs of Excessive Pronation
- Posterior Tibial Strength
- External Hip Rotator Strength
- AJDF (looking for equinus forces)

Common Mechanical Changes for Medial Knee Compartment Syndrome (with the common ones used in RED)

1. Valgus Wedges
2. Orthotic Devices Preventing Supination
3. Varus Wedges
4. Orthotic Devices Preventing Pronation
5. Knee Braces (General and Off Loading)
6. Quadriceps Strengthening
7. Hip Strengthening
8. Shock Absorption Inserts (custom Hannafords, etc.)
9. Training Techniques for Increase Knee Bend
10. Shoe Selection

Valgus Wedges are really the mainstay of treatment of medial knee compartment syndrome. Their mechanical function is to open up the medial compartment. The valgus wedge is utilized to open up the medial compartment and shift more weight to the lateral compartment. Typically, you are allowing the foot to pronate more, but preventing or postponing medial meniscus or knee replacement surgeries. The complexity is in deciding who is a candidate for valgus wedging and how much. Patients with normal knee mechanics really do well with valgus wedging. Patients with lateral instability do well, but could need a lot of wedging to achieve the goal of less knee pain. Patients with excessive foot pronation most likely will require a varus wedge, but the rules here seem 50/50. Valgus wedges tend to be ¼ inch heel wedges, or ⅛ to ¼ inch lateral foot wedges. The wedges can be free standing, glued to the shoe insert, placed into the midsole of the foot, or placed as a lateral outsole wedge about 1 inch in width.

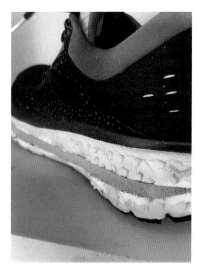

Valgus wedge placed as a Shoe Midsole Wedge

Orthotic Devices Preventing Supination function as huge valgus wedges in the patient with contact or propulsive phase supination. Their mechanical function is to prevent medial compression from foot supination at contact, but indirectly make the lower extremity so much more stable. It is the heel supination that crowds the medial knee compartment. It is up to the prescribing provider to decide what should be in this orthotic device. The basic ingredients: 1) a suspension or computer scanned mold if the patient has an everted forefoot deformity, 2) correction around heel vertical or slightly everted, 3) lateral Kirby Skive, 4) high lateral heel cups or phalanges, 5) Denton Modification, 6) Forefoot valgus forefoot extension, 7) Feehery Modification, or 8) Cuboid Support.

Practical Biomechanics Question #386: The motion of the knee joint is both simple and complex. Since the motion of the knee joint is influenced by 3 areas, how it responds to

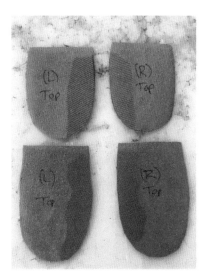

Grinding Rubber from JMS Plastic used for Varus or Valgus Wedges

a certain treatment may not be predictable. What are the 3 primary areas that affect knee motion? Answer: 695

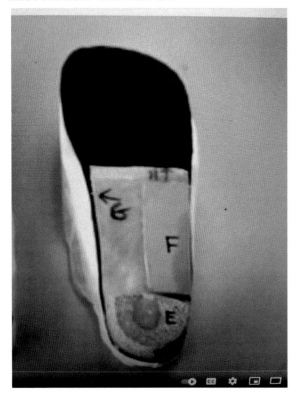

Denton Modification is vital for supination control is marked "F" here

Varus Wedges are used when medial knee pain is typically not from rearfoot supination and subsequent overcrowding, but pronation as discussed above can cause some medial compartment compression at times. Their mechanical functions are usually at stabilizing the knee by decreasing the medial position of the knee over the foot and making the foot more stable. There are times when the knee is unstable, or at least made more stable with varus wedges to control pronatory instabilities. When I am put to the task of designing shoe wedges or other inserts to help with knee pain, I first must decide on varus, valgus, or a straight heel lift. If my first guess is incorrect, and

the symptoms worsen or just do not improve, I try the other techniques. I simply explain to the patient that I am trying to find a place in the knee that is healthy to take the majority of pressure. The valgus wedge pushes the weight bearing laterally, a varus wedge pushes the weight bearing medially, and a heel lift shifts the weight forward. Like valgus wedges mentioned above, they can be stand alone, or applied to the midsole or outsole of the shoe.

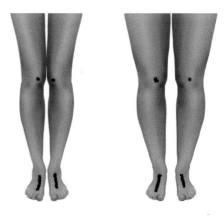

Here the Internal Position of the Knee can be helped with varus wedging of the foot

Orthotic Devices Preventing Pronation are discussed in the orthotic device chapter ahead in Book 4. The mechanical function is to make the foot and knee more stable. The less the foot is pronated, the more stable the bone structure becomes. Also, as the diagram above shows, incases of excessive internal positioning of the knee, varus wedges and custom orthotic devices, can dramatically improve alignment. The typical components utilized are: 1) balancing of forefoot deformities when using a Root device, 2) deep heel cups, 3) medial phalanges, 4) heel inversion by some method (straight cast inversion, Kirby skives, or Inverted technique), 5) rearfoot posts and anterior posts, and 6) forefoot varus forefoot extensions. When dealing with the knee, the more rearfoot correction of pronation control the better.

Knee Braces (General and Off Loading) are normally for the orthopedist to decide, but sometimes I have to bring up the subject. Their mechanical function is to provide light compression and support to the musculature. Patients can get simple wrap around ones that can instantly add stability. I typically point them in the right direction, and then can ask their orthopod for a more exact recommendation.

Practical Biomechanics Question #387: Braces cause a positive biofeedback loop. Braces cause proprioceptive awareness while wearing. Explain how this proprioceptive awareness can help in the injury rehabilitation. Answer: 695

Practical Biomechanics Question #388: How does one normally avoid the negative effect of braces which can cause us to lose muscle while wearing them? A:695

Quadriceps Strengthening is both quad sets (isometric) and single leg presses, but the knee can be challenged with single leg raises and short arc squats. Their mechanical function is to take stress away from the joint. These are 4 easy quadricep exercises that can be done early in the rehabilitation process well before the patient can get to the physical therapist.

Practical Biomechanical Question #389: Name four simple but effective knee strengthening exercises that Podiatrists can start the patient on while waiting to begin Physical Therapy treatment? Answer: 695

Hip Strengthening can be for the general purpose of strengthening the proximal muscle group to take pressure off the knee in general. And, in acute injuries, strengthening the knee at a certain point in time will be too painful, and strengthening the hip will get the rehabilitation plan going. Therefore, their mechanical function concerns off weighting the knee joint by the more proximal strength, and attempting to directly strengthen the muscles to change bad positions. Hip strengthening can be very specific also to help control either pronatory (internal) or supinatory (external) forces, along with hyper-extension or flexion forces..

Shock Absorption Inserts (including custom Hannafords, etc.) have to be tried with any form of knee, hip or low back arthralgias. Their mechanical function is to lower the impact shock that goes into the knee joint. I love Spenco for its shock absorption properties as a straight heel or full length insert. I love plastazote and poron combinations also. If I wanted to make a custom orthotic device for mainly shock absorption, it would be the Hannaford technique.

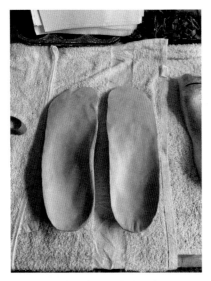

Pair of Hannafords with leather top cover

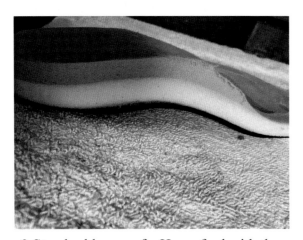

3 Standard layers of a Hannaford with the softest plastazote against the skin (bought JMS Plastics in New Jersey)

Training Techniques for Increase Knee Bend is standard for patients that lock their knees. Their mechanical function is to directly decrease stress at the knee joint and place it onto the soft tissue. The mantra is to "make your knees softer" with a slight knee bent with prolonged standing. Sometimes this means for them to run with a lower center of mass dropping the pelvis and bending their knees.

Shoe Selection requires typically 3 points:

1. Some heel height to help with knee bend
2. A more neutral shoe with no tendency to supinate the foot
3. A soft cushion insole and midsole for better shock absorption

However, when pronation can be blamed on the pain, getting into a more stable (stability) shoe may be the best option. This is when experimenting with what makes the knee feel better initially. Do you find it varus wedging or valgus wedging brings the most relief? Then you can tailor your shoe recommendations to fighting supination or pronation. If either feel better at the knee, you can try flat soled non heeled shoes vs shoes with heel raise (called zero drop vs more traditional heels shoes).

Lateral Knee Compartment Syndrome

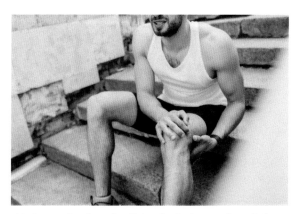

Pain at the level of the inferior pole of the Kneecap remaining lateral to that point may be lateral knee compartment syndrome

Of the two knee compartment syndromes (medial and lateral), this is the easier for podiatrists to wrap their heads around. And, in general, the general rule is true. What is the general rule? The general rule with lateral knee compartment syndrome is to varus wedge the foot. Placing a varus force at the foot, transfers the weight at the knee more medially, and opens up the lateral joint line. It is very effective, for both attempting to avoid surgery, or eliminate pain after surgery. It was for lateral knee compartment syndrome that I first started using the Inverted Orthotic Technique. It is a solid principle, and you can off load the lateral knee joint. Yet, it takes work by the referring orthopod, the patient, and the varus wedging podiatrist. Too much causes problems, too little does not work (like a bandaid to a laceration).

To tie this into Chapter 3 and 4 on gait and biomechanical examination, with lateral knee compartment syndrome, we are looking for signs of pronation that causes compression forces that we can fix, and the most important examinations to do in 10 minutes (or 20 minutes) are:

- Signs of excessive pronation in gait
- Genu Valgum in Stance
- RCSP
- NCSP
- Quadriceps and External Hip Rotator weakness
- Poor Shock Absorption

Common Mechanical Changes for Lateral Knee Compartment Syndrome (with the common ones used in RED)

1. Varus Wedges
2. Orthotic Devices with Varus Tilts
3. Knee and Hip Strengthening
4. Knee and Hip Flexibility Program
5. Shock Absorption Insoles and Shoes
6. Hannaford Custom Orthotic Devices
7. Knee Braces Including Off Loading
8. Gait Training
9. Technique or Training Changes

Varus Wedges are really the hallmark of treatment a podiatrist does to help lateral knee joint issues, or the Occam's Razor for this problem. Their mechanical function is to open up the lateral knee joint taking pressure off of the compartment. The knee joint motion is really influenced by foot motion, knee joint motion, and hip motion. Varus wedges are therefore one third of the approach, but can be the most important aspect of the knee treatment both conservatively, and even post-surgical. I have been honored by working side by side with orthopedists my whole career, some who want my direct involvement in their knee care, and some we just share patients by location. However the situation, I have been able to treat knees from the foot standpoint for years and have had incredible results. Varus Wedges can be applied as a stand alone heel wedge, a wedge applied to the shoe insole, a wedge applied to the midsole of the shoe, and a wedge applied to the outsole of some shoes. The goal of varus wedges is to increase weight to the medial side of the knee and open up the lateral joint line. Typically, I work in the ¼ to 3/16 inch range.

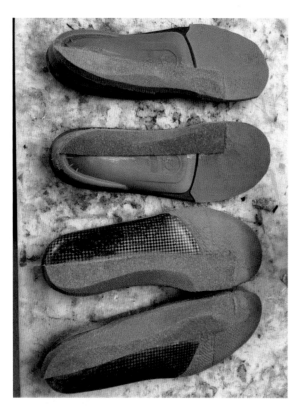

Here Varus Wedges of ¼ inch Grinding Rubber from JMS Plastics applied to various OTC arch supports for a patient

Orthotic Devices with Varus Tilts really started with inverting Root Balanced orthotic devices and varus wedging shoes to get the rest of the force. Their mechanical function was to open up the lateral knee joint line and decrease compression forces. The rule was not to invert a Root Device more than 3 degrees, so you had to get more varus support from elsewhere. First, it was the Inverted Orthotic Technique, which Chapter 13 will discuss, then it was the Kirby medial heel skive, and combinations of the two. Orthotic Laboratories across the country started experimenting with more and more inversion into the correction (probably up to 10 degrees that I have seen).

Practical Biomechanics Question #390: As we place a varus correction at the foot in an attempt to open up the lateral knee joint, what muscles must we strengthen to protect against overdoing it? Answer: 695

Knee and Hip Strengthening are crucial to provide external support to the knee. Their mechanical function is to directly or indirectly stabilize the knee. In general, a physical therapist directs a non painful program to strengthen the 2 main motions at the knee and the 6 main motions at the hip. Based on the patient's unique biomechanics, individual muscle groups may be more important like the external hip rotators when there is excessive internal knee rotation. It is crucial to make patients more stable in the process of a generalized program. Many patients are also too loose, and this leads to problems like knee hyper-extension. Selective muscle strengthening can be very useful. I use hamstring strengthening routinely in my patients that tend to hyper-extend their knees as one example.

Knee and Hip Flexibility Program is maintaining or establishing normal joint flexibility. Their mechanical function is to decrease abnormal positional changes due to the tight muscle groups. Again, the physical therapist tends to look for tightness in the 2 knee and 6 hip muscle groups. It is rare that you want anything too tight, but based on the patient's unique biomechanics, one muscle group may be the most important to work on. In the case of lateral knee compartment problems, you should definitely work on lateral hamstring, lateral knee fascia, iliotibial band, and lateral quadriceps flexibility. Think about it from the tightness side of the problem. If all four of those structures are tight, then any of them can abnormally compress the lateral knee joint line.

Shock Absorption Insoles and Shoes make sense when you are trying to decrease the shock into an injured knee caused by ground reactive forces. Their mechanical function is to decrease shock entering the knee from ground impact. I prefer Spenco products, but there are many on the market that do the trick. The opposite is what you have to, even more importantly, be aware of making heel contact too hard. I have switched patients with hip and knee joint arthralgias into softer shoes, softer orthotic devices, or just modified their current devices to make the heel softer. This has to be balanced with an eye on stability as more cushion can mean more instability. At times the maximalist shoes, like Hoka One One, make sense for the cushion, but they do change heel strike patterns so more caution is warranted.

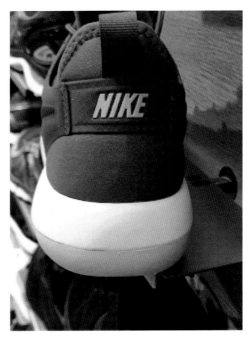

One of the definitions I like for maximalist shoes is that the midsole looks like it does not belong on the shoe.

Hannaford Custom Orthotic Devices represent a soft custom made functional orthotic device. Their mechanical function is extremely soft or shock absorbing, but very stable, therefore decreasing the stress across the knee joint. Their weak link is in the durability. Most podiatrists have their favorite version of soft based orthosis, but I encourage them to learn Hannaford and compare. Designed by Dr. David Hannaford, this is an incredible device for shock absorption, and can be wedged or other forms of modifications. There is something simple in treating patients with a pure shock absorbing device with arthralgias complaints.

Practical Biomechanics Question #391: Working with Hannaford for the last 35 years has taught me most of their uses. They are the king of Shock Absorption. Why were they originally designed for runners?

Knee Braces Including Off Loading typically prescribed by the orthopedist and physical therapist, but many times in my practice I was the one who recommended it. Their mechanical function is to stabilize and off load at times. Any treatment modality for any patient may prove to be the most significant one. Simple knee braces, which add support and warmth to the area, can be miraculous.

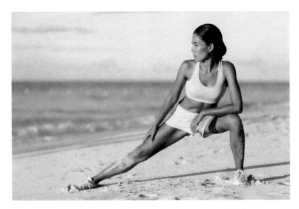

Simple Hip Adductor Stretch which would place too much valgus compression across the lateral knee joint line

Gait Training for lateral knee compression forces is basically narrower your gait to get the weight more medial, or to bend your knees to prevent extension forces. Its mechanical function is to recognize gait patterns that can be changed that can alleviate stress on the lateral knee joint. It is during gait training that the physical therapist may pick up on the over pronation forces that need a varus wedge, or hyper-extension forces that need more knee bend.

Technique or Training Changes is where the Athletic Trainer or Physical Therapist looks at all aspects of their workouts and determines if changes in knee extension or lateral knee stress can be made. Of course, it may start with just slowing everything down. Then you want to look where the knee is too straight, or goes into knee valgus positions. Can these be changed?

Pes Anserinus Syndrome

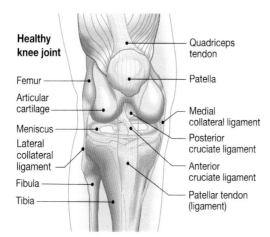

General Anterior Knee Anatomy with the Pes Anserinus attaching Medial to the Patellar Tendon to stabilize the that area

The powerful pes anserinus (meaning "goose feet") attaches on the anterior medial tibial plafond and acts to stabilize the forward motion of the tibia in stress situations like running downhill. When you land at foot strike (foot contact), the tibia moves forward and is naturally internally rotating with foot pronation to dissipate forces. The pes anserinus attachment is meant to stabilize that motion from going too far with the combined fibres of the sartorius (hip flexor), gracilis (adductor) and the semitendinosus (hamstring). The mnemonic used to remember these 3 is SGT (sargeant). It is also protecting the ACL who shares that function among others. Pes Anserinus tendinitis or bursitis is most commonly seen in runners with a history of downhill use. Along with iliotibial band syndrome, it is a running related injury, meaning you typically only see them in runners. You should be somewhat suspicious for another problem when a

non-runner presents with pes anserinus pain.

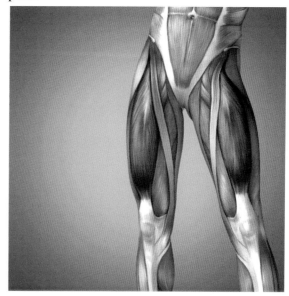

The fibres from the Sartorius and Gracilis are seen making up part of the Pes Anserinus on the Medial Aspect of the Proximal Tibia

To tie this into Chapter 3 and 4 on gait and biomechanical examination, with pes anserinus syndrome, and the most important examinations to do in 10 minutes (or 20 minutes) are:

- Running Gait Evaluation for signs of overpronation
- Walking Gait Evaluation for signs of overpronation
- Static biomechanical examination tests looking at pronatory causes that can be treated (like forefoot varus)
- Muscle testing of muscles that resist pronation (external hip rotators, posterior tibial, etc.)

Common Mechanical Changes for Pes Anserinus Syndrome (with the common ones used in RED)

1. Avoiding downhill running until symptoms have resolved
2. Knee Braces
3. Knee Taping
4. Varus Wedges
5. Orthotic Devices with Added Pronation Control
6. Shoe Changes
7. Muscle Strengthening Exercises
8. Muscle Flexibility Exercises
9. Gait Training
10. Cross Training

Avoiding downhill running until symptoms have resolved is some of the best advice you can give with runners, if they can still run some, or if they are just starting to run again. Its mechanical function is to decrease the stress at the anteromedial knee. As you run downhill, the pes anserinus has to work incredibly hard to prevent you from falling forward by shoring up the anterior medial knee. This is especially true in overpronators who are already stressing this area with excessive internal knee rotation and knee flexion.

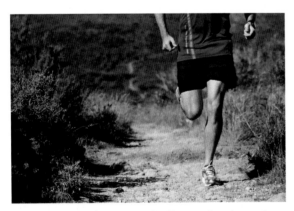

The Stress after Foot Strike at the Anterior Medial Aspect is magnified running downhill and the knee is supported by many muscles including the Pes Anserinus

Knee Braces can be simple reinforcements to the anterior knee and play a role in allowing a return to activity sooner than without the brace. Their mechanical function is extra support to the anteromedial knee area. I have good luck in the many simple over the counter braces you get from sporting good stores. I typically leave the recommendation to their physical therapist or orthopedist for a more exact recommendation since there are so many braces on the market. Patients with pes anserinus bursitis at the insertion may not like the pressure from the brace and prefer taping.

Knee Taping may not be as supportive as a brace, but can be much more comfortable, and more directed to the function required in general based on the amount of sensitivity. Their mechanical function is to stabilize the anteromedial knee joint line.

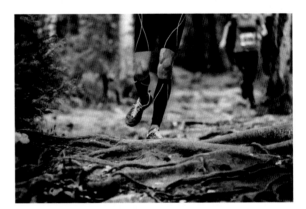

Here knee taping is utilized to stabilize the anterior aspect of the knee reducing stress on the pes anserinus

Varus Wedges are a common method of bolstering up the medial anterior side of the knee. Their mechanical function is to indirectly stabilize the anteromedial knee area. The wedges are typically ¼ inch and primarily the heel only when walking. Wedges can be increased to either midfoot or sulcus length when the pronation force is later in the gait cycle. All of my athletes with pes anserinus problems get full length varus wedges to protect them when they are on the ball of the foot.

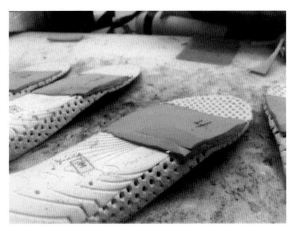

Here forefoot strikers get the varus wedging (thicker on the medial side) at the ball of the foot

Practical Biomechanics Question #392: Medial or varus wedging of the foot can have a great effect on pes anserinus problems. When would you make the wedge longer than just a heel wedge? A: 695

Orthotic Devices with Added Pronation Control is related to the point of foot strike in runners. Their mechanical function is to decrease the internal torque on the anterior medial aspect of the knee. Runners have 3 distinct landing patterns: heel strike, midfoot strike, and forefoot strike. Controlling the area involved in the landing is crucial in treatment. The rearfoot strikers need more rearfoot control, the midfoot strikers more midfoot control, and the forefoot strikers more forefoot control. With rearfoot strike, techniques like the Inverted Orthotic Device or the Kirby Skive make sense. With Midfoot Strike, orthotic devices with good medial arch support are crucial. With Forefoot Strike patients, the addition of forefoot wedges or extensions made in varus are the most important aspect.

Practical Biomechanics Question #393: Explain why the control of pronation can differ in orthotic design between various runners based on their strike patterns. A:696

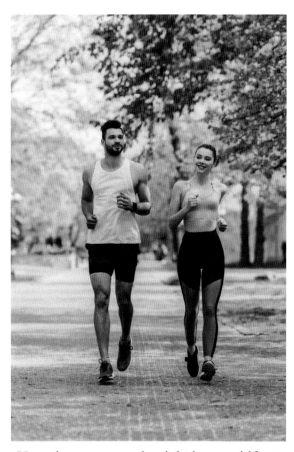

Here the runner on the right has a midfoot land and the runner on the left a heel strike pattern. Orthotic devices for runners must consider this strike pattern

Shoe Changes to a more stable shoe is important in decelerating the amount of contact phase pronation which is their ideal mechanical function. However, the fit across the midfoot is crucial for ideal support. This can mean a narrower and shorter shoe than ideally fits can be better as a general rule. Also, lacing techniques like "power lacing" are crucial to lock down the heel and midfoot areas.

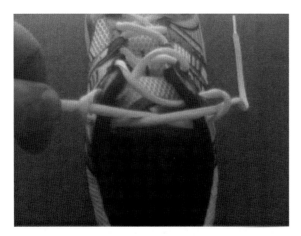

Power Lacing is crucial when you use orthotic devices to prevent the instability caused by any heel slippage

Muscle Strengthening Exercises for any muscle that decelerates pronation and stabilizes the anterior medial aspect of the knee are important. This is the mechanical function of these exercises. Of course, the three muscles that make up the pes anserinus should all be strengthened: sartorius, gracilis, and semitendinosus. This is an anatomical masterpiece. These 3 muscles, parts of 3 separate muscle groups, are used for the powerful function of stabilizing the knee joint.

Practical Biomechanics Question #394: What 3 muscle groups make up the pes anserinus? Answer: 696

Muscle Flexibility Exercises should definitely work on hamstring flexibility if the knee is too flexed, and therefore unstable by nature. The mechanical functions of muscle flexibility exercises are typically 2 fold: taking tendon off the knee is some way, and decreasing the tension which leads to over pronation syndrome. Tightness also makes tendons less strong, so any muscle/tendon that is too tight around the hip, knee, or ankle could potentially cause a weakest issue. Tight external hip rotators, like the piriformis, can hold the knee too external, and not in line with the internally rotating foot at heel strike. Tight internal hip rotators, like the adductors mainly, can hold the knee too internally rotated and not centered over the foot well in activities.

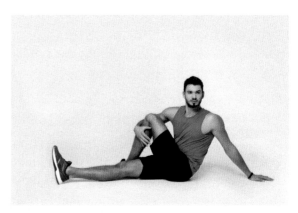

Classic Piriformis (External Hip Rotator) Stretch

Gait Training can be utilized to decrease the torque at the knee. Its mechanical function is to change the stresses across the injured area, initially almost completely, and then the stresses can be slowly added back to the athlete's workout. Definitely, keeping the runners off the downhill for a while while they rehabilitate makes sense.

Cross Training can be used to stay in shape while you are injured in the short term, and long term to strengthen but minimize the overuse of running every day. Its mechanical function is to keep the injured area strong, the surrounded areas strong, and overall physical fitness in as good condition as possible

Lower Hamstring Strain

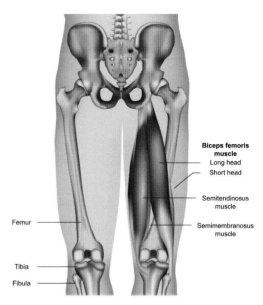

The Medial and Lateral Hamstrings behind the thigh and then crossing the knee

The hamstrings are powerful muscles with their tendons in the back part of the thigh crossing the knee joint. They are divided into both medial and lateral, and into lower and upper. The medial hamstrings are the semimembranosus and semitendinosus (which we just talked about as part of the pes anserinus). The lateral hamstrings are the long and short heads of the biceps femoris. It is important for biomechanics whether the hamstrings are too tight (holding the knee too flexed), or too weak (upsetting the delicate quadriceps to hamstring balance) which allows for too much knee extension and hyper-extension. The hamstrings can be tight in the lower part only, upper part only, or both, so patients have to learn how to stretch both the upper and lower parts of the hamstring. Sciatica, or more likely radicular nerve pain, can masquerade as tight hamstrings with hamstring pain with quite different treatments. The hamstrings also can just be too weak. There is a delicate 50% balance between quadriceps and hamstrings with the hamstrings being 50% weaker for daily living, and closer to 80% in athletic endeavors. This is important since the quadriceps at foot strike play an important role in preventing the knee from flexing too much and the patient landing on their face (or some other body part). The tighter the hamstring, the weaker the hamstring as taught to us by force length curve physics. Plus, the more flexed the knees stay, the more unstable the knees are and more prone to injury. I have to make sure the reader understands that the calf, quads, and hamstrings are primarily sagittal plane (straight line) movers. This is important when the rotational forces in the frontal or transverse planes predominate around the knee. When these sagittal plane movers have to move slightly twisted, they can strain more. This is why pronation (placing the knee too internal) and supination (placing the knee too external) with its transverse plane excessive motions, or high degrees of coxa vara or coxa valga, genu varum or genu valgum, can be stressful for the hamstrings. Overall, we can not forget that the role of the quadriceps and hamstrings (with some help from the popliteus, iliotibial band, and pes anserinus) protect your knees. Therefore, anything off (alignment issues, rotational issues, weakness or tightness issues) can make their job harder thus injuring the knee joint easier. Our job as Podiatrists is to lower the

risk at the knee for injury by reducing obvious problems we see.

To tie this into Chapter 3 and 4 on gait and biomechanical examination, with lower hamstring strain the most important examinations to do in 10 minutes (or 20 minutes) are:

- Pronatory signs in gait and exam
- Supinatory signs in gait and exam
- Limb Length Discrepancy signs in gait and exam
- AJDF for equinus forces or over stretched achilles
- Hamstring and Quadriceps Strength and Flexibility

Practical Biomechanics Question #395: What is the classic mechanical reason why a weaker than normal hamstring muscle can cause knee pain? Answer: 696

Common Mechanical Changes for Lower Hamstring Strain (with the common ones used in RED)

1. Achilles Flexibility
2. Hamstring Flexibility
3. Quadriceps Flexibility
4. Hamstring Strength
5. Quadriceps Strength
6. Short Leg Treatment
7. Correction of Pronatory Forces
8. Correction of Supinatory Forces
9. Cross Training
10. Training Changes
11. Taping

Achilles Flexibility is one of the first contributions podiatrists can add to the treatment of this problem. The mechanical function is to specifically decrease the knee flexion caused by a tight gastrocnemius muscle. A tight gastrocnemius causes increased knee flexion and allows for both the knee instability and the reason the hamstrings begin to tighten. Therefore, the mechanical function of achilles flexibility is to correct any tightness found in the gastrocnemius which could lead to knee instability.

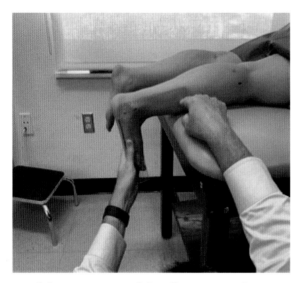

Measurement of the Gastrocnemius Flexibility with the Knee Straight (see Chapter 4 for the exact measurement technique)

Hamstring Flexibility is vital to most hamstring strains, and almost all knee problems. Its mechanical function is to prevent a tight hamstring from being easily stressed. When the hamstring is too tight, the knee is bent and relatively more unstable and prone to injury. The general rules of stretching will be outlined in chapter 11 of Book 3 and the hamstrings are one of the funnest to try all the principles to get them stretched out. Since you have both the lower and upper hamstrings, along with the medial and lateral hamstrings, there are

typically 4-6 stretches that make up a good hamstring stretching program.

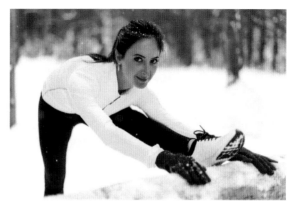

Athlete stretching the lower hamstrings

Quadriceps Flexibility is one of those crucial areas, but an indirect cause of hamstring issues. The mechanical function is to allow ease of knee flexion caused by the hamstrings. The tighter the quadriceps are, the more strain on the hamstrings to bend the knee. This is similar to anterior shin splints with tight achilles tendons. The tighter the achilles, the harder the ankle extensors have to flex an extended ankle. They have to pull up against gravity anyway, and the tight achilles, like a heavy shoe, can just be the breaking point. The vastus lateralis is the tightness of most quadriceps, so quadriceps stretching should be done with the opposite hand pulling the foot upwards and backwards. The goal is typically to pull the foot away from the body, not just pull up to touch the buttock.

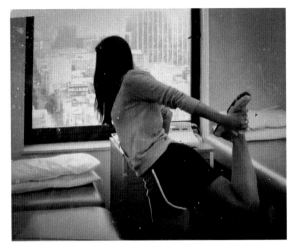

Quadriceps Stretching done correctly with opposite hand on foot and foot pulled backwards and upwards

Hamstring Strength has always been a huge issue. The mechanical function is that the weaker the tissue and more easily it will strain. The delicate balance of hamstring to quadriceps strength is vital at around 60-80% (with the quadriceps being stronger). Definitely, with hamstring strains, you want more of an 100% ratio of equal strength like in anterior cruciate ligament tear rehabilitation. These numbers are typically obtained in a 1 Rep Max Test, or by the comfort limits of a patient doing their hamstring curls.

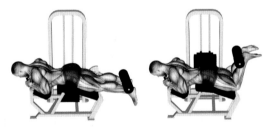

Hamstring Curls

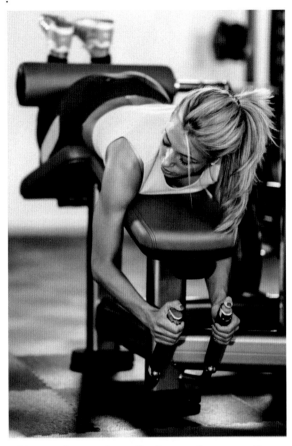

Hamstring or Leg Curls are done at a Set Weight

Quadriceps Strength in hamstring strains is typically stronger than hamstring strength in the delicate H/Q Ratio. The mechanical function of strengthening the quadriceps is to make the knee more stable. A stable knee is going to put less strain on the muscles that guard it. I prefer a single leg press to achieve my quadriceps strength, but there are many ways of strengthening this muscle group.

Practical Biomechanics Question #396: When would you prescribe a double leg press versus a single leg press? Answer: 696

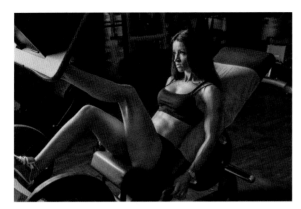

Single Leg Press

Short Leg Treatment is an area I spend a lot of time analyzing with hamstring strains. The mechanical function of lifts in treating a short leg can help level the stresses equally on the two legs. There are many possible issues that we deal with in terms of having a leg length discrepancy. I refer the reader to my chapter upcoming on leg length difference and its treatment. First, the spinal tilt caused by the leg length difference can put more pressure on one leg over another. This is called leg dominance and there is more stress on the dominant side. Secondly, the normal compensation for a long leg is the body's attempt to shorten the long leg. How is this done? The long leg pronates more at the subtalar joint and flexes the knee. Both the abnormal pronation stresses the hamstring (typically forcing it to function out of the sagittal plane), and the increased knee flexion causes hamstring tightness. The resultant hamstring tightness causes relative weakness and strain. And there is stress to the hamstrings due to the tightness directly.

Correction of Pronatory Forces is important in the hamstring rehabilitation of a pronator, or someone with chronic hamstring issues and the problem of over pronation. The mechanical function will be either direct by making the knee more stable, or indirect, by making the lower extremity more stable. You are always decreasing knee flexion which helps hamstring issues. The hamstrings are sagittal plane movers, so the twists or rotational torques and moments of force produced by over pronation can be a reason for chronic strain. Review Chapter 5 in Book 2 as it discusses all the treatments of pronation from simple to complex. The patients will give you feedback as to whether a treatment is helping their problem, although in this situation you are still making the patient more stable by eliminating some or all of the pronatory forces.

Correction of Supinatory Forces is due to the hyper-extension of the knee produced by excessive rearfoot supination. That is the mechanical function of correcting rear foot supination. If normal pronation is allowed, then some normal contact phase knee flexion will occur (relaxing the hamstrings). When the foot hits the ground, the knee should gently flex as the foot pronates. This knee flexion is replaced by a knee extension force (when the foot supinates instead of pronates) that puts a strain on the hamstrings.

Cross Training is a nice way to take tension off the hamstrings when they are injured. The mechanical function of cross training is to decrease the stress through the hamstrings while during the early phases of rehabilitation. Swimming overall is a nice stretch to the hamstrings, and adjusting the seat height to a stationary bike can be raised or lowered until the hamstrings feel better. It is so crucial to keep moving, as rest itself just tights up the tissue more. Moving slow initially is better than fast, and some lessening of impact is preferred.

Training Changes uses the same principles as cross training, but allows the sport to continue. A runner may have to lessen the hills, slow the pace, or do some walk-run alternating program.

Taping is generally with Kinesio Tape (or one of the other flexible tapes) and meant to keep the knee slightly flexed. Its mechanical function is to add both stability and flexion in cases of hyper-extension stresses.

Practical Biomechanics Question #397: I repeat over and over to the students I teach that their treatment of knee, hip and low back problems can be very crucial. What are the 2 main reasons foot over pronation can produce lower hamstring pain? A: 696

Practical Biomechanics Question #398: What does subtalar joint supination do at the knee joint closed kinetic chain? A: 696

Practical Biomechanics Question #399: In Chapter 1 Book 1 the concept of Rule of 3 was introduced. It basically means that 3 different potential causes of an injury can create the "Perfect Storm" and the injury occurs. Explain 3 or 4 reasons why a patient in an overuse situation can develop lower hamstring pain. Answer: 696

Iliotibial Band Syndrome

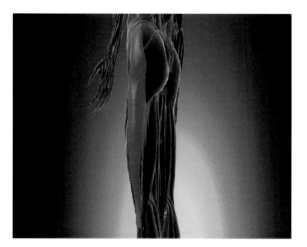

Iliotibial Band course from pelvic to tibia

The iliotibial band is a dense ligament that is formed by the fibers of the tensor fascia lata anteriorly and the gluteus medialis posteriorly. The IT Band runs from the iliac crest at the pelvis to Gerdy's tubercle on the anterior lateral tibia between the head of the fibula and the tibial tuberosity. Its main function is to stabilize the lateral aspect of the knee and hip at heel contact. Since its demands are so much greater in running (imagine protecting the hip as you land running fast down a hill), it is typically a running related injury, like pes anserinus tendinitis or bursitis. The literature well documents that this problem is related to overpronation where the band rubs across either the greater trochanter near the hip, or the lateral femoral epicondyle by the knee. These motions of irritation following heel contact are from posterior to anterior as the fibula internally rotates faster than the femur, while the subtalar joint pronates.

Yet, in my practice, I have found two other causes that frequently cause iliotibial band syndrome. Short leg syndrome typically means we are not perfectly stacked straight and have some limb dominance (side lean) with motion. Imagine if the Leaning Tower of Pisa had iliotibial bands and how stressed they would be all day trying to right the ship. I find in cases of bilateral iliotibial band syndrome that limb difference is important to correct. I find with unilateral iliotibial that the long or short leg can be individually involved.

I also find that excessive supination, yes the polar opposite of over pronation, can cause iliotibial band syndrome. The excessive supination produces lateral instability (or just lateral overload to the limb) which stresses the lateral structures of our feet, ankles, legs, and thighs. It is easy to imagine how an iliotibial band strain can arise from over-supination. It definitely occurs more, or isolated to, in the more supinated foot.

To tie this into Chapter 3 and 4 on gait and biomechanical examination, with iliotibial band pain with are looking for signs of supination which can cause lateral overload the lateral column, or pronatory signs that may indicate excessive torque, or signs of short leg syndrome, and the most important examinations to do in 10 minutes (or 20 minutes) are:

- Running Gait Signs of Overpronation
- Running Gait Signs of Oversupination
- Running Gait Signs of Limb Length Discrepancy
- Limb Length Difference Measurements
- RCSP
- NCSP
- Static Measurements of Pronatory Signs
- Static Measurements of Supinatory Signs

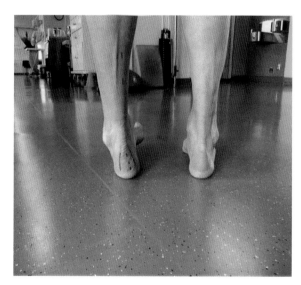
More Supinated left foot from behind

Common Mechanical Changes for Iliotibial Band Syndrome (with the common ones used in RED)

1. Stretching
2. Strengthening
3. Correction of Abnormal Pronation
4. Correction of Abnormal Supination
5. Correction of Short Leg Syndrome
6. Taping
7. Shoe Change
8. Training Modification

Stretching of the iliotibial band is somewhat controversial, like stretching the plantar fascia, but patients express such great improvement in symptoms. Its mechanical function is to decrease stress in especially the bands that are very tight. There are many ways to stretch, and please review the upcoming chapter on stretching principles. I am attaching my own YouTube stretching video for the iliotibial band to review here. https://youtu.be/rI1uUQv7u1k

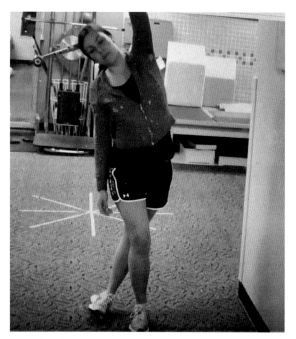

Windmill Stretch demonstrated for the left IT Band (the left foot must be inverted)

Strengthening of the hip abductors is crucial in the rehabilitation of the iliotibial band. Its mechanical function is to keep the tone in the injured area, especially when localized weakness is part of the problem. The photo below shows the classic hip abduction against gravity. You can eventually use resistance bands when 2 sets of 25 active ranges of motion is easy. Please see the general comments in the chapter on weak muscles on how to progress through your strengthening program later in this book.

Practical Biomechanics Question #400: With the main function of the iliotibial band to stabilize the lateral side of both the knee and hip, it is easy to see how injuries occur. In a patient with limb dominance to the left, what side would tend to develop IT Band symptoms? Answer: 696

Also vital in the treatment of iliotibial band syndrome is the recognition of over pronation or over supination. In the overpronators, the external hip rotators are crucial to strengthen. In the supinators, the hip internal rotators and adductors and medial hamstrings are important to strengthen.

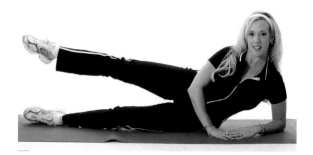

Hip Abductor Strengthening

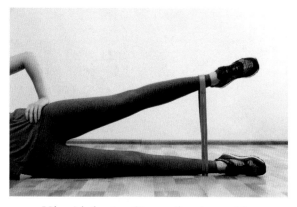

Hip Abductor Strengthening with Resistance

Correction of Abnormal Pronation is initiated after watching the patient run (if they are a runner), or walk (if they do not run) and determining that the patient has abnormal pronation as a possible cause. Its mechanical function is to decrease the transverse plane torque across the knee and hip. Typically the patient is told to get more supportive shoes (stability over neutral), given ¼ inch varus wedges or OTC inserts to begin the process of pronation control.

Correction of Abnormal Supination occurs when the patient exhibits over supination in gait. Its main mechanical function is to decrease the lateral stress of the lower extremity. Since this is primarily a running injury, valgus wedges free standing or glued to the bottom of the shoe insole are initiated. For all runners and all injuries, you must direct the correction where they strike or land: rearfoot, midfoot, or forefoot. This should influence where the wedging occurs.

Correction of Short Leg Syndrome is initiated when limb dominance, a gait sign of short leg syndrome, is noted. Its mechanical function is to reduce the side lean caused by limb dominance. The patient is like the Leaning Tower of Pisa with the iliotibial bands attempting to right the ship. For so many runners that spend most of the time up on the forefoot, heel lifts do not help, or as much, as full length lifts. See the upcoming chapter on limb length discrepancy.

Taping is normally for pronators to stop the pronators for an anterior to posterior

Iliotibial Band excursion. Its mechanical functions are for support and reduction of anterior movement over the lateral bony prominences. But, I have seen lately, much more only lateral tissue reinforcement .

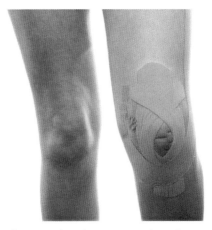

Quite Involved Knee Taping for PFD and IT Band

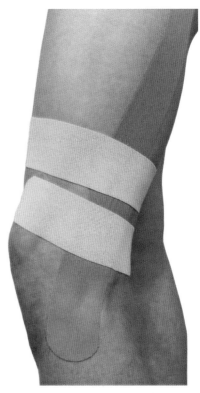

IT Band Reinforcement with Blue and Green pulled anterior to posterior with some tension

Shoe Change is necessary for 3 mechanical objectives. The first is you just may change the shoe to more cushion to help the knee joint stress (an indirect cause of iliotibial band, but a direct cause of problems like joint arthralgias or tibia and femoral stress fractures). Secondly, you may change the shoe for better pronation control in a pronator. Those dealing with pronation with orthotic devices and stability shoes do have to be careful not to overdo it and turn a pronator into a supinator. Thirdly, shoes can be used to help over supination, which is sometimes called underpronation, when this lateral instability or lateral overload is considered the cause of iliotibial band tendonitis. There are fewer of these stable, but neutral shoes on the market currently like the Saucony Triumph, New Balance 1540, Adidas NMD, or Brooks Ghost.

Training Modification is initially just trying to decrease the activities that cause pain, or decrease the range of knee motion if walking even hurts. Its mechanical functions are to allow activities with less stress to the healing tissue. Adding cross training to the normal routine is next, and cycling tends to give the best workout for injured runners. Swimming is also a favorite. Finally, training modification occurs if activities that caused initial symptoms are gradually and slowly introduced back. If the patient is a pronator, then activities like downhill running can be the last added to the increased pronation (which also gives pes anserinus symptoms). It can be a great adventure discovering which activities increase pronation or supination, and how those activities can be modified.

Practical Biomechanics Question #401: Why do women tend to get IT band symptoms more at the hip than men? (696)

Femoral Stress Fractures

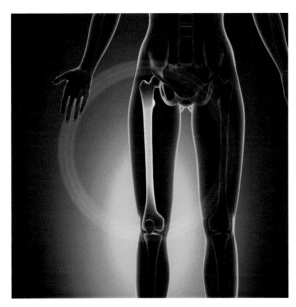

Femur Highlighted

Podiatrists can provide a wonderful role in the treatment of athletic produced femoral stress fractures. In fact, my first case of using my beloved Hannaford orthotic device, the master of shock absorption, was a runner with repeated femoral stress fractures around 17 miles in training for a 26 mile marathon. And, each femoral stress fracture was in a different place, and each with possible serious consequences. With the Hannaford, and the added shock absorption they provided, she ran 7 marathons in the next 10 years until I lost track of her. Is it always shock absorption problems that cause femoral stress fractures, probably not, but they are the only ones I have had the privilege to treat. We have talked about poor shock absorption, but what are the treatable components?
They include:

- Excessive loading with increased miles, especially downhills
- Functioning in a maximally pronated position (need the motion of pronation for shock absorption), or in contact phase supination (same reason)
- Limited subtalar joint motion (rigid foot)
- Running technique with too much heel jarring
- Running with excessive pronatory torque
- Shoes that are too hard

And, if we add poor bone health, from transient low Vitamin D, to more slowly changing Low Bone Density, we are set up for femoral stress fractures.

One of the problems with treating femoral stress fractures is that you are not treating pain at present. The femur breaks and the patient is taken through the phases of rehabilitation. As podiatrists, we are taught, and I emphasize, that we look for the cause for possible reversal, not just treat the symptoms. The cause is poor mechanics, something that makes it more prone to break, and these can be intrinsic to the bone, extrinsic to the bone, or both. Intrinsic would be bone health, and extrinsic would be poor shock absorption or excessive pronatory torque.

To tie this into Chapter 3 and 4 on gait and biomechanical examination, with femoral stress fractures the most important examinations to do in 10 minutes (or 20 minutes) are:

- Signs of Poor Shock Absorption
- Signs of Rigidity

- Signs of Maximal Pronation or Contact Phase Supination
- Signs of Excessive Rotational Pronatory Torque with Running
- RCSP
- Forefoot Deformities
- Subtalar Joint Range of Motion

Common Mechanical Changes of Femoral Stress Fractures (with the common ones used in RED)

1. Varus Wedging
2. Inverted Orthotic Devices if Significant Pronation Running
3. Training Modifications
4. Reversing Supination
5. Increase Shock Absorption
6. Muscle Strengthening
7. Shoe Modifications

   Varus Wedging is a simple way to begin to correct over pronation which may or may not be related to the specific problem. Its mechanical function is to reduce the pronatory torque on the femur, or to enable the subtalar joint to get out of a maximally pronated position. In a pronator, you must get a feel for abnormal and dangerous or mild and an annoyance, to know when to treat. One of my golden rules of practice is to always make the patient more stable. It applies in all cases, as you must create rules that seem to work. In pronators, called medial instability patients, varus wedging makes them more stable. The varus wedges for a runner typically goes anteriorly under the big toe joint medially and is between ¼ inch and ⅜ inch, and can be very soft as the image below where I have made the varus wedges out of poron material. Runners must

be controlled in the forefoot, as well as the rearfoot, as they will spend probably half of their time running on the front of their foot. This is especially pertinent in forefoot strikers.

Practical Biomechanics Question #402: We have long known in medicine that fractures can be produced by excessive pounding and by rotatory torque placed on the bone. Explain several other factors related to bone injuries that are common problems. A: 697

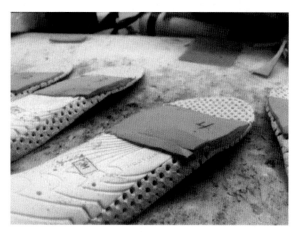

In a Forefoot striker (landing point) the Varus Wedging (thicker under the big toe joint side) must be at the Forefoot

   Inverted Orthotic Devices if Significant Pronation While Running can be the only way to capture the excessive pronation moments or torques. This is a custom made varus wedge of sorts. Its mechanical function is the same as a varus wedge just mentioned allowing for more shock absorption and total foot contact. You are balancing control of rotational forces with shock absorption when dealing with stress fractures. After a femoral stress fracture has been rested (Immobilization Phase of Rehabilitation), and I can begin to allow a Walk Run Program (see chapter on Office Handouts) in the Return to Activity Phase, I typically use a Hannaford style orthotic device and varus wedge that, or press the Hannaford off an Inverted cast. That way I have both the stability and shock absorption.

Training Modifications can be both temporary as you build the ability to handle running stress back up, or more permanent as you discuss with the patient how they train. Its mechanical function is to allow tissue to heal by reducing the shock the body has to absorb. The excessive shock or rotatory torque with pronation may be fixed primarily with shoes and inserts allowing return to pre-injury levels, but it may be that the majority of abnormal forces lie in the training itself. Patients can typically get addicted to their programs and forget to have enough recovery time. This is why we build 48 hours of recovery into the early rehabilitation programs. Yet, the actual workouts can be modified in the short and long runs, including less downhill running, putting the downhill aspect of the workout at the beginning of the run, switching to quality workouts over straight distance every time, running hard uphills but slow downhills, etc. Of course, training modifications can mean permanent cross training which runners initially fight, but thank you for in the long run. Early in the injury rehabilitation, cross training is a crucial way to increase activity when running is either non-existent or at low mileage. Typically cross training only lowers the impact shock so cycling, swimming, and elliptical are fine. I think the stair master has too much force on the femurs to be part of a cross training program for femoral stress fractures. As running is allowed again, encourage your athletes to choose softer surfaces to start. And, ideally, attempt to change a hard heel striker, into a midfoot or forefoot striker.

Practical Biomechanics Question #403: Why is switching from running down hills at the end of runs to the beginning of runs helpful for femoral and most stress fractures? Answer: 697

Reversing Supination can be crucial in femoral stress fractures, hip arthralgia, sacro-iliac and low back issues. Its mechanical function is to help a patient pronate which is great for shock absorption. If patients come in with any of these problems, and I can correlate them to over supination gait patterns, I know I am going to be successful. Contact phase pronation allows for shock absorption. Contact phase supination prevents some, if not all, of the limb's shock absorption, and stress fractures can occur. I refer you to the custom orthotic chapter on excessive supination treatment at the start of Book 4. But, simply a $\frac{1}{8}$ to $\frac{1}{4}$ inch valgus wedge attached to the shoe insert in supinators may be all you need.

Increase Shock Absorption is the obvious treatment of femoral stress fractures. Its mechanical function is self explanatory. This can be running on softer surfaces, insoles with Spenco or Poron, and Hannaford custom devices.

Muscle Strengthening is a vital part of every rehabilitation program including femoral stress fractures. Its mechanical function is to allow the muscles to take the stress from the bone. Here we need the quadriceps and the hamstrings to take load away from the femur. This is why cross training is vital, especially cycling which develops these muscle groups. The stronger the muscle, the less stress on the underlying bone. Also, strengthening both distal and proximal muscles from an injury (foot/ankle and core in this case) can help take stress off the injured area significantly. I discuss with patients routinely with foot injuries that by strengthening their core they are lifted off their feet. I like that mental image.

Shoe Modifications is a reminder to look at the shoes they were wearing when injured and see if the basic style can be improved. Their mechanical function is to add more shock absorption or prevent excessive rotatory torque. Do they need just more shock absorption? This of course typically gives them a little more instability. Or, if they are wearing shoes that seem soft and stable, the Brooks Ghost and Adrenaline come to mind, perhaps just alternating shoes, like alternating workouts is best. I love patients to run with several pairs of shoes each giving different stresses almost every other time they run. It is in running daily with the same shoe with its same stresses that injuries can occur. But, with shoe rotations, the variation of stress can be wonderful in avoiding some repetitive use injuries. However, I still think this is only a part, and recovery time is crucial.

Hip Joint Arthralgias

As a podiatrist, I treat hip pain indirectly. The patient is seeing a doctor and a physical therapist either at the same time which is ideal, or me alone due to their current foot problem. I weekly get the patient who was told to come back to the hip surgeon when they are ready for a hip replacement only. No rehabilitation is offered at all. Of course, this makes my job easier. Patients are aware that the foot can cause hip pain. When I see a patient with hip and low back pain, leg length discrepancy is on the top of my mind. If you watch someone walk, and they land harder on one side (called limb dominance), they probably have a leg length difference to treat. You can order a Standing AP Pelvis X-ray barefoot in a normal stance to get an exact measurement of their overall leg length difference, and some impression on how healthy the hip joints are. I refer you to the upcoming chapter on leg length difference. However, both shock absorption issues can jar the hip joint causing pain, or hip range of motion problems can cause jamming of the hip joint and resulting pain. This will be discussed further in a second.

It is important to discuss both referred pain and what I call "tip of the iceberg" pain. Referred pain is commonly related to the hip. The hip may hurt, but the problem is being referred from the knee or low back or the sacro-iliac joint. The low back or knee may hurt only, but the real problem comes from the hip. So, referred pain has to be considered in any hip, knee, or low back workup. Tip of the Iceberg pain is where the pain presently is really only a sign of a bigger problem below the water. Many patients present with some form or another of hip strain or bursitis, only to have a bigger problem of hip arthritis or femoral stress fracture discovered in the workup or follow up visits.

To tie this into Chapter 3 and 4 on gait and biomechanical examination, with hip joint arthralgias the most important examinations to do in 10 minutes (or 20 minutes) are:

- Signs in Gait of Short Leg Syndrome
- Limb Length Discrepancy Examination
- Signs in Gait of Poor Shock Absorption
- RCSP
- Signs in Gait of Hip Hike or Stress
- Hip range of motion examination

Common Mechanical Changes for Hip Joint Arthralgias (with the common ones used in RED)

1. Limb Length Discrepancy correction
2. Shock Absorption Orthotic Correction
3. Training Modification
4. Varus Wedges with Pronation
5. Valgus Wedges with Supination
6. Shoe Modifications
7. Strengthening Exercises
8. Stretching Exercises

Limb Length Discrepancy correction is explored in greater detail in Chapter 10. Its mechanical function is to even the stress through the hip joints in weight bearing. Correcting for short leg syndrome is a valuable part of my practice and the treatment for hip arthralgias. As you watch the patient walk, with limb length discrepancy, one leg will be dominant. That means the body is compressing that side more with greater trunk mass over the hip socket. In adults, the dominant is typically the longer side, so putting more pressure gradually on the short side by the use of lifts can be very helpful. With each step, you can take 10-20% stress off of the sore hip. It is trickier to treat when patients fall to their short leg when that is the painful hip. You still have to add the lift to the short side gradually, however that can increase the pressure on the sore hip initially increasing pain. I advise the patients with this scenario, that the hip should feel better when the weight distribution gets close to even. Over a quarter inch difference then makes it hard, and I sometimes skip the breakin and the typical gradual progression of lifts.

Practical Biomechanics Question #404: When standing with a quarter inch short right leg, what leg would you typically lean on when there is no pain? Answer: 697

Shock Absorption Orthotic Correction makes sense with any joint arthralgias, especially the hip. Its mechanical function is to decrease stress of impact at the hip joint. The hip joint responds well to more shock absorption whether it is coming from lessened impact in activity, softer surfaces, shoes, soft inserts, and custom orthotic devices designed for better shock absorption. The three main functional focus points of orthotic devices to add to a patient's improvement in shock absorption

are: better cushion at the point of impact (varies for walking vs running landing positions like rearfoot strike or forefoot strike), reversal of contact phase supination (we need contact phase pronation for shock absorption), and enhanced rearfoot pronation (especially when maximally pronated throughout gait). This can be simply setting the foot slightly inverted and letting it pronate to the ground with a flexible plastic, or grinding motion into an extrinsic rearfoot post. I think the Hannaford custom orthotic device (and most labs have a version) will easily help you achieve a custom effect of total foot contact to spread the weight evenly out to the entire foot, and provide incredible shock absorption in the plastazote layered material utilized. Ask your orthotic laboratory what version they make for maximum shock absorption while maintaining stability.

Practical Biomechanics Question #405: Why does increasing pronation at heel contact help in shock absorption in the leg?

Training Modification typically means less impact, so more cycling, elliptical, swimming, and other activities. Its mechanical function is to lessen the stress at the hip joints. When running is allowed, start with slower speeds and minimal to no downhill running. Less heel impact shock is crucial, so learning more midfoot to forefoot running is encouraged. As runners attempt more speed, they can make the mistake of over striding with more exaggerated heel contact and overall lower extremity shock that needs to be absorbed by the tissues. Even doing more speed work, instead of doing long slow distance, can help.

Varus Wedges with Pronation is a common treatment for hip arthralgias if you recognize more pronatory torque, especially with rapid internal femoral rotation. Its mechanical function is to slow down hip rotation, but also prevent the hip joint from reaching its end range of internal rotation motion. There is more chance of hip injury when the internal pronatory rotation forced by the foot is more than the internal rotation of the hip itself. If you see a lot of internal rotation in gait, but not a lot in static examination, this problem may be occurring, and varus wedges tend to be a great solution.

Practical Biomechanics Question #406: What motion of the hip is decelerated, or reduced, when applying a varus wedge under the heel in the shoe? A: 697

Valgus Wedges with Supination is very common in my practice. The patient presents with hip pain and excessive contact phase supination is noted. Its mechanical function is to attempt to produce contact phase pronation vital for shock absorption. This supination at the subtalar joint hyperextends the knee and places a vertical jolt to the hip joint, or the sacro-iliac joint. There can be tremendous sophistication dealing with over-supination which will be discussed in the upcoming orthotic chapter, however a simple ⅛ to ¼ inch valgus wedge (free standing or attached to the shoe insole) can be a very powerful first step. This mechanical change is also sometimes more

diagnostic than x rays or MRIs if it leads to a great reduction of symptoms. We need contact phase pronation and this is what our goal is to create with the valgus wedges.

Practical Biomechanics Question #407: Why is hip joint pain sometimes helped with varus wedges, and sometimes with valgus wedges? Answer: 697

Shoe Modifications should correlate to what you are trying to accomplish from our discussion from above: more shock absorption, more pronation control, or more supination control. These are the mechanical functions of shoes. Yet, for a lot of problems including hip arthralgias, and with the type of orthotic device the patient wears, you may find that the orthotic device gives the pronation or supination control so the shoe only needs to add some shock absorption. Or, you may have the orthotic device, like my beloved Hannafords, give the shock absorption and the shoe must give the frontal plane support. It is a fun area to experiment with especially with the patients pre- or post- hip surgeries (attempting to prevent or speed their recovery) as they are a dedicated group. Even though I have not come to any conclusions, it seems that the zero drop shoes straighten the knee at impact and increase the stress on the hip joint. Yet, it may be the opposite, as zero drop shoes seem to allow better full foot strike with less knee and hip stress. It is great to have your patients rotate their shoes to vary stresses anyway, so they may be able to tell you which shoe type gives the best hip relief.

Strengthening Exercises really can be the entire chain of lower extremity muscles up to the core. The mechanical function concerns muscle strengthening will take stress off the bones and joints in the area. Specifically, you should generally strengthen the 6 hip muscle groups: adductors, abductors, flexors, extensors, internal rotators and external rotators. After the hip, it is important to strengthen above and below the hip joint, therefore low back and knee. As you assess the patient's biomechanics, it may be important to strengthen an unstable ankle, a weaker opposite leg, or the anti-pronation or anti-supination muscles. This would be based on your judgment of what is causing stress to the hips. A lack of internal hip rotation with over pronation tendencies can be helped with supinatory corrections at the foot level to prevent the hip from internally rotating so far as one example.

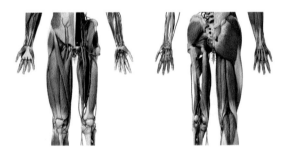
Anatomy of Hip Muscles

Practical Biomechanics Question #408: Name muscles that help prevent excessive foot pronation motions that could jam the hip joint into a maximally internal rotated position. Answer: 697

Stretching Exercises for the 6 hip muscle groups are intellectually simple, but can create a challenge with hip arthralgia patients. Why is this the case? Muscles tighten to protect, muscles tighten due to nerve hyper innervation, and muscles feel tight when they are just strains or overworked. The mechanical function of hip stretches is to relax tension in overly tight muscles. Hip arthralgia patients need to learn the basic hip stretches, but should be warned to never stretch through pain and if they hurt more after stretching you have to know. Sometimes it takes a patient to break down the stretches to a different one each session to learn which one is painful. Sometimes tight muscles are good due to their protective function, so stretching them out is actually the wrong idea. But, all in all, if the patient does stretching and feels better, you are probably on the right course. The hip in general functions the best in the middle of its range of motion, so measure the range, see if they seem to be in the right spot, or have them stretch to get better. If they are too internal, those are the muscles to stretch while you strengthen the external hip rotators. If they are too external, stretch the external while you strengthen the internal hip rotators..

Upper Hamstring Strain

The upper part of the hamstrings gives you that pain near the buttock that is often sciatic nerve related. It is much harder than the lower hamstrings to help since muscles are harder to stretch than tendons. These injuries are at or near the insertion into the ischial tuberosity (your "sit" bone). Anyone that treats the achilles knows it is easier to treat the body of the tendon by appropriate stretches, than the attachment into the heel bone. Insertional hamstring strains are more like enthesopathies with an element of tendonitis, periosteal reaction and bone inflammation. The hamstrings, divided into the medial and lateral parts, are both internal rotators and external rotators along with their function of knee flexion. And, to make things more challenging, the hamstrings assist in terminal extension of the knee (last 5 degrees or so). Therefore, the treatment of hamstring strains has to consider how the knee is being internally rotated too much (strain on the lateral hamstrings, and produced by tightness to the medial hamstring), or being externally rotated too much (strain on the medial hamstring, and produced by tightness to the lateral hamstrings), or extended too much (stress on both hamstrings), or flexed too much (how my sitting position here typing for long periods is producing tightening of both hamstrings). Oftentimes, the upper or lower hamstrings only strain in acute injuries, so the cause is known, and the subtleties are in the rehabilitation. Oftentimes, the hamstrings develop soreness in overuse situations, and a greater understanding of their overall function with the rest of the lower extremity, potential tightness, or relative weakness, is crucial. And finally, hamstring strain that does not respond to treatment, maybe all sciatic nerve tension. The appropriate treatment here is less hamstring and more nerve focused.

To tie this into Chapter 3 and 4 on gait and biomechanical examination, with upper hamstring strain, the most important examinations to do in 10 minutes (or 20 minutes) are:

- Signs of Over Pronation
- Signs of Over Supination
- Hamstring Strength and Flexibility Measures
- Signs of Gait Problems with the Knee Too Straight or Flexed

Common Mechanical Changes for Upper Hamstring Strain (with the common ones used in RED)

1. Upper Hamstring Stretches (different than lower hamstring)
2. Strengthening
3. Neural Flossing or Gliding
4. Avoid Sitting for prolonged periods
5. Varus Wedges for Over Pronation
6. Valgus Wedges for Over Supination
7. Heel Lifts
8. Shoe Modifications
9. Compression Sleeves or Hose
10. Training Modifications

Practical Biomechanics Question #409: Upper Hamstring problems can be sciatic nerve problems in disguise. Explain the comment test for sciatic nerve symptoms.

Upper Hamstring Stretches (different from lower hamstring) have to be done supine with the hip flexed as far as possible without lifting the pelvis off the table and slowly straightening the knee. Their mechanical function is to ease the strain produced by tight hamstring muscles. Some patients simply lie on the floor and put their straight leg up a wall, but it is not as good. https://youtu.be/KEFpJaMwEtQ This video demonstrates upper vs lower hamstring stretches.

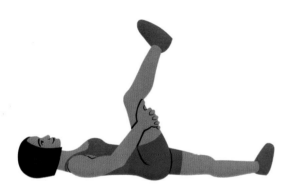

HAMSTRING STRETCH

Typically the flexed hip is maintained while the knee is straightened by a wall or towel wrapped around the foot. You have to start this exercise with the knee bent to take the lower hamstring out of the equation.

Strengthening of the hamstrings is typically with lower leg curls, although this is better for lower hamstring strength. Its mechanical function is to keep the tone and strength in the stressed tissue. If the muscle/tendon gets too weak with the injury, it will be vulnerable for repeated injuries or delayed healing. This seems to be quite normal in hamstring injuries. Since most patients do not have access to the gym readily, simply progressing through initially active range of motion, isometric, and progressive resistance exercises can get the patient started. Isotonic with weight progression can begin a month or so later under the guidance of a physical therapist or personal trainer.

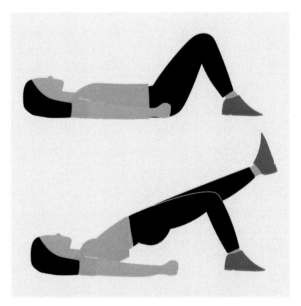

This single leg Bridge is a beginning isometric shown for the right side. Count for 20 seconds and repeat three times. I prefer the right heel in this image to be on the ground only (not the whole foot).

Neural Flossing or Gliding is a great exercise for the sciatic nerve. Its mechanical function here is to keep the nerve calmed down, so muscle rehabilitation can continue. It is a rhythmic motion of gentle flexions and extensions of the lower extremity. It is great if some of the hamstring problems are rooted in neural tension. It can also help in diagnosis based on how it makes the patient feel (much better or worse in sciatic nerve problems).

Many subtle sciatic nerve conditions do not have positive straight leg tests. Therefore, neural flossing can bring your attention to the problem being more a nerve issue, or just make the hamstring feel more comfortable when there are neural tension issues co-existing. I have attached a video showing one of the flossing routines https://youtu.be/g94F8g_jzGg.

Avoid Sitting for prolonged periods is a general rule for all hamstring issues. Its mechanical function is to decrease the compression on the hamstring origin at the ischial tuberosities "sit bones". The hamstrings can get really tight when they are flexed in the sitting position for long periods of time. The upper hamstring particularly gets compressed by the chair while sitting. Some doctors or therapists recommend sitting on a physioball for some time each day or getting a standing desk to avoid the compression aspect of this injury.

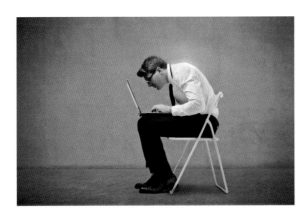

Prolonged sitting can irritate the upper hamstrings at their origin at the ischial tuberosities

Varus Wedges for Over Pronation of ¼ inch are typically used in patients whom excessively pronate with upper hamstring

strain. Their mechanical function is to decrease transverse plane rotatory torque. These are a bit tricky since they are primarily heel lifts which can increase knee flexion also. As I will talk about in a minute, the increased knee flexion can tighten the hamstrings making matters worse, or relax the hamstrings when the knee is too straight making matters better. But, all in all, it is good to see if it helps at least in the short term.

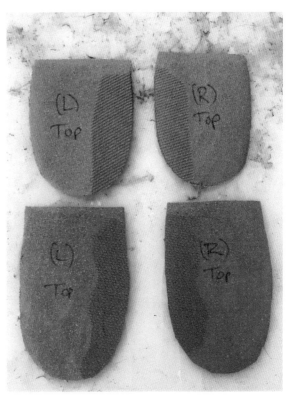

Varus Wedges of different lengths (can also be valgus wedges for supinators)

Valgus Wedges for Over Supination are also ¼ inch and primarily heel modifications and lifts. It is used in patients that over supinate at heel contact. Its mechanical function is to flex an over extended knee. Supination will cause knee extension, so you are not only reducing a transverse plane rotational component, but you will be flexing the knee as just discussed.

Heel Lifts can be a vital treatment for upper or lower hamstring problems. As with achilles issues, in the short term, heel lifts should simply take tension off the hamstrings by slightly flexing the knee.This is its mechanical function. In the long run, heel lifts can add to knee tightness if the patient is not educated on hamstring stretching. You may initially need up to ½ inch of heel lift to help the patient, and remember to place the same amount on the uninvolved side. As the patient gets better, you will then need to gradually reduce the lifts so as to not get too radical a change at once. Therefore, a ½ inch goes to ⅜ inch, then a ¼ inch, then ⅛ inch, and finally no lift. If the patient is not coming into the office with this regularity, then multiple lifts have to be given and carefully marked to guide this progression from home.

Shoe Modifications are primarily (mechanical function) to change the heel lift or height based on what success has been found with heel lifts. You can advise the patient to stay flat (now called zero drop), or to increase the shoe's heel height to well over ½ inch in some running shoes (16 mm is the highest I have heard). In general, the higher the heel the better with hamstring injuries, unless instability is created like in a 3 or more inch dress heel. That leaves us with the second mechanical function of shoes which helps with pronation or supination stability as needed per patient.

Compression Sleeves or Hose or Shorts can provide external support and warmth to these injuries. I am attaching the website of one of my favorite companies. https://110playharder.com/ Their mechanical function is in slight stability, and also warmth to the tissue.

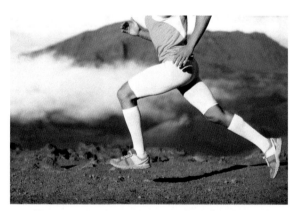

Extra tight support for Upper Hamstring injury for warmth and slight support

Training Modifications are really based on the severity and level of recovery. Their mechanical function has to fit with the Phase of Rehabilitation. Remember, hamstrings are basically sagittal or straight

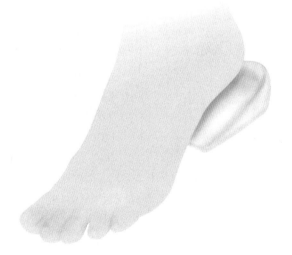

Heel Lift added to both feet

moving muscles, along with the quadriceps and achilles. Therefore, you can allow straight ahead slow walking then running first, before rotational activities. The basic cross training with cycling, elliptical, and swimming normally are fine, but occasionally if the knee is too bent (cycling) or too straight (elliptical), symptoms will flare. I know the basics, but tend to leave this to our physical therapists or athletic trainers.

Practical Biomechanics Question #410: What is the position of the knee at the time of an acute injury to the lower hamstring versus the upper hamstring? A: 697

Piriformis Syndrome

When someone walks or runs, the piriformis is a muscle meant to initially decelerate internal hip rotation, and then externally rotate the hip and thigh in midstance and propulsion. It has to work harder when we overpronate, since over-pronation forces it to fire elongated and work harder decelerating the internal femoral rotation. Yet, it is the piriformis muscle in relationship to the sciatic nerve that really gives us our major problem. The sciatic nerve runs above, below, or right through the muscle in some people. The nerve can get irritated in some way by the excessive motions of the piriformis. Piriformis syndrome can give you classic sciatica or just various other nerve symptoms that can be hard to find the cause of down the chain. It is typically in correcting excessive pronation that helps piriformis syndrome, although there are other causes. .

To tie this into Chapter 3 and 4 on gait and biomechanical examination, with piriformis pain we are looking for pronatory signs that make indicate excessive torque, and the most important examinations to do in 10 minutes (or 20 minutes) are:

- Signs of Excessive Pronation In Gait
- Signs of Excessive Pronation in Stance Measurements

Common Mechanical Changes for Piriformis Syndrome (with the common ones used in RED)

1. Varus Wedges
2. Shoe Modifications

3. Neural Flossing or Gliding 3 times daily
4. Piriformis stretching
5. External Hip Rotation Strengthening
6. Sciatic Nerve Guidance

Varus Wedges are the primary method that podiatrists use to help patients with many problems, including piriformis. Their mechanical function is to slow down excessive pronatory rotation of the lower extremity. If the piriformis muscle is fatiguing trying to slow down contact phase internal femoral rotation associated with over pronation, then ¼ to ⅜ inch varus wedges can work magic. And, a slight change in the foot, due to a long lever arm, can produce a big change at the knee and hip. It is the general rule that if you change the foot ¼ that you may change the hip ½. This is more or less in individuals, but the patients can grasp the significance of what you are attempting to accomplish. See the image of these varus wedges, that can be made full length also, in the last section on Upper Hamstrings. Vaurs wedges can not only be inserts, but midsole wedging or outsole wedging.

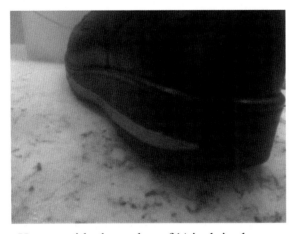

Here a midsole wedge of ¼ inch is shown

Shoe Modifications are typically more stabilizing for the pronator. Their mechanical function is the same as varus wedges to slow down pronatory (internal) rotation of the lower extremity. Every activity can need a stable shoe and stable insert (custom or customized OTC). Also included here are various other means of stability including: varus wedges to the midsole of the athletic shoe, power lacing, lacing over velcro enclosures, and proper fit to the heel and midfoot to avoid the foot moving in the shoe.

Neural Flossing or Gliding 3 times daily like with Upper Hamstring problems can be diagnostic for nerve issues. Their mechanical function can be to separate out nerve problems from muscular problems. Piriformis Syndrome can give a variety of nerve symptoms. There can just be nerve symptoms, along with musculo-skeletal symptoms that need to be separated and improved upon. As a patient is flossing or gliding the nerves, if the symptoms get either better or worse, you are demonstrating that the baseline problem is a nerve issue. With nerve issues, you want a good referral source to a local neurologist or physiatrist.

Piriformis stretching is helpful when the muscle gets tight, and then clamps down hard on the sciatic nerve. The mechanical function of piriformis stretching is to relax the external hip rotator by internally rotating. There is a lot of discussion as to the correct way to stretch. The image below shows a classic piriformis stretch. However, the piriformis becomes an internal hip rotator due to a change in its axis as you flex the hip. However, this is a very common stretch that seems very helpful.

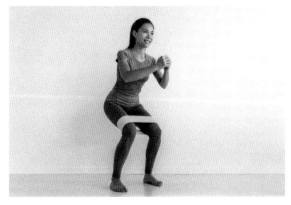

Here is a standard piriformis strengthening exercise. From the position shown, the knees are externally rotated against the resistance of the band.

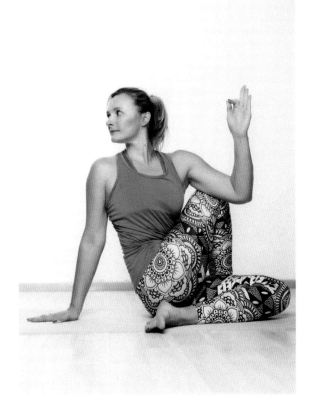

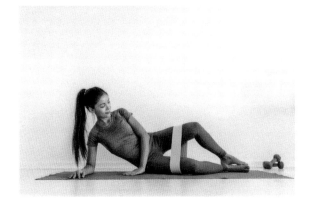

Similar exercise to strengthen the Piriformis. You start with the knees together, with band resistance you externally rotate your hips to separate the knees.

Strengthening the piriformis can not be isolated from the other external hip rotators: gluteus medius, gluteus minimus, obturators, piriformis, sartorius, and tensor fascia latae. Its mechanical function is to make sure the piriformis is strong in activity and less likely to strain. It is important that the knee is not flexed, or there can be too much torque injuring the knee while doing these exercises.

Sciatic Nerve Guidance is typically given by a physical therapist to my patients. When the sciatic nerve is involved in piriformis syndrome, it is so important not to keep irritating the nerve. Its mechanical function is to separate out nerves from muscle involvement. The classic issues of minimal hip bending, keeping the knees bent while lifting, and not going into full ankle dorsiflexion are commonly heard from our physical therapists. I want them to discuss with my patients how the sciatic nerve gets irritated on a routine basis so that the patient does not keep aggravating the problem. Physical Therapists in the Association of Neurologic Physical Therapy become a good find for the piriformis patients when there is nerve involvement.

Practical Biomechanics Question #411: Explain the concept of Triple Crush on the nervous system in a piriformis patient that overly pronates, hyper-extends her knees while standing at work, and stretches her achilles by standing off the end of her stairs.

Practical Biomechanics Question #412: Explain how this exercise (shown below) may put stress on the sciatic nerve. A: 698

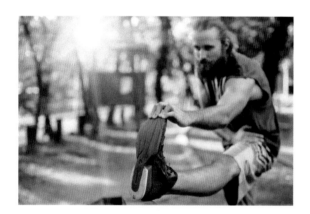

Sacroiliac Pain

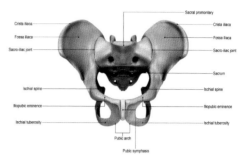

Female Pelvis: Anterior view

The sacroiliac joint glides inferior-superior and can get jammed up or down. The joint feels sore when it gets irritated, and many times it is hard to differentiate from low back causes, or even hip issues. I have seen the mechanical causes of sacro-iliac pain develop when there is a short leg syndrome and when the foot overly supinates. As we get higher up the chain away from the foot, I understand my knowledge of the SI joint is fairly limited. But, when you are treating problems in the lower extremity, patients will comment whether the treatment helped or irritated their sacro-iliac joints. When there is a need for lift therapy, at the same time there is an unstable SI joint, your treatment may fail because the sacro-iliac joint will go out of place in the loading from the lift, before you can level the pelvis. Treating hip and low back pain from a podiatrist's standpoint has been incredibly rewarding and sometimes very frustrating. I tell my students at the California School of Podiatric Medicine to never shy away from trying to make someone more stable (or level in this situation). It may be the best treatment ever given to the patient. Where I have similar stories in this area, I will save Ben's story for the section on low back pain.

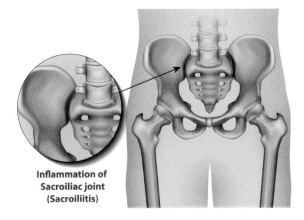

Inflammation of
Sacroiliac joint
(Sacroiliitis)

Sacro-iliac pain presents more like back pain then hip pain. I would say of my patients with "back" pain, many prove to have just SI joint pain. As we watch patients walk to get an idea of their biomechanics, at times we see the sacro-iliac joint (at S2 spine level) jerk up and down, or an asymmetry in the motion between the two sides. As we stand the patient, we are all taught to palpate 3 pelvic landmarks in our limb length difference evaluation: ASIS, PSIS, and Iliac Crests. Not only are you looking for one side higher, but you are looking for the common signs that the pelvis is off: one side looks higher on one or two but not all three landmarks, one side looks more forward, or one side looks further away from the midline. This gives you some idea that a referral to a physical therapist or low back specialist is in order. Then, when you lay the patient supine, look at the position of the feet from you. While the patient is standing, you are getting a reference of the pelvis to the ground, but while the patient is lying you are getting a reference to the pelvis to the low back. In general, they can be opposites, so one practitioner calling the right leg shorter, and another (using another set of landmarks) calling the left leg shorter, is not an unusual occurrence.

When we watch a patient walk, if there is a lean consistently to one side, it is called limb dominance. Most of the time, adults fall to the long leg which jams up the sacro-iliac joint on that side. Children, and young adults to 30 or so, can be 50/50 which leg that they fall towards. Let us say that this is the left side that is long. When this common occurrence is assessed by standing the left side appears higher, and when this common occurrence is assessed lying supine the left side will appear the short side as the compression forces to their long side sacro-iliac jams the joint upwards. The left foot will be further away from you.

To tie this into Chapter 3 and 4 on gait and biomechanical examination, with sacro-iliac pain, the most important examinations to do in 10 minutes (or 20 minutes) are:

- Limb Length Discrepancy Evaluation
- Gait Evaluation for LLD signs
- Gait and Static Evaluations looking for Asymmetries
- Gait and Static Examination for Excessive Supination Tendencies

Common Mechanical Changes for Sacroiliac Pain (with the common ones used in RED)

1. Stretching Exercises

2. Strengthening Exercises
3. Lifts for Short Leg
4. Valgus Wedges for Supination
5. Varus Wedges for Pronation
6. Self Reduction Exercises
7. Shoe Changes

Stretching Exercises are a vital part of sacro-iliac pain to relieve tension. The mechanical functions appear to be two-fold: release tight musculature and help push or pull a jammed SI joint back towards its neutral place. As a podiatrist, I typically cotreat these patients with an MD and physical therapist and leave the exact exercise to them. I have been personally plagued with right sided sacro-ilac pain due to a dorsally subluxed SI joint (originally a basketball injury from being undercut and landing hard on my right foot with my knee extended pushing the ilium to the upper part of the sacro-iliac joint). The stretches I do will be different when dealing with pain from another cause. Like piriformis and upper hamstring pain, a component of nerve pain can be masked as joint pain. If the stretching exercises you are given tend to make things feel worse, question the basic diagnosis as the nerve system tends not to like prolonged stretching.

Strengthening Exercises that are pain-free can be started within days or hours of your injury. Their mechanical function is for stabilization of the sacro-iliac joint and low back. For the purpose of this book, this should be left to the MD and physical therapist team. Since sacro-iliac joint pain can be recurrent, you want to develop 4 or 5 maintenance home exercises for pelvic and low back stability. Since so many patients have a very unstable pelvis by history, they should be strengthening the surrounding muscles daily. The 4 exercises I always want patients to work on: hip adduction, hip abduction, bridging, and the bird dog pose from Yoga.

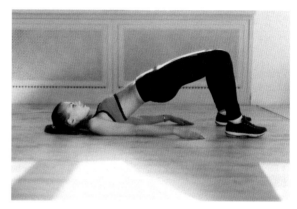

The Bridge hold is gradually increased based on strength and pain development

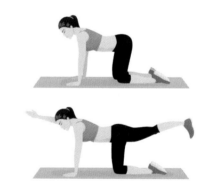

Bird Dog Pose is done with opposite legs and arms (and both sides)

Lifts for Short Leg is my contribution to typically chronic sacro-iliac pain. Their mechanical function is to attempt to even the stress across the SI joints. See the chapter coming up on common thoughts to short leg treatment. If the side that the patient falls to when walking (limb dominance) is the side of the sacro-iliac pain, negating the limb dominance with lifts tends to help. My first thought when the SI joint pain is on the opposite side of the limb dominance, so less weight bearing pressure, that I better have nerve pain higher in my differential. Compression forces on one side of the disc caused by limb dominance can allow the disc to bulge on the opposite non-compressed side. Subtle differences of even ⅛ inch over someone's lifetime, or over the course of training for the Olympics or a marathon, can cause symptoms to develop.

Valgus Wedges for Supination can be effective at ⅛ inch or greater when excessive supination is noted in gait. Their mechanical function is to allow contact phase pronation easing stress on the SI joint. Valgus wedges can be simple inserts in the heel or full foot, midsole wedges, outsole wedges, or part of a custom orthotic device. The cause may be simply corrected with a custom orthotic device in the long run which I prefer. Custom foot orthotics can be designed like the concept of total contact casting for diabetics. The idea is to distribute the weight evenly to the whole foot as you are correcting supination or pronation tendencies. Excessive contact phase supination straightens the knee when it should be flexing and places an upward jamming force across the knee, hip, and SI joint. The knee straightening effect also pulls on the hamstrings increasing low back pain as it straightens the lumbar curve from its neutral position. With a straighter lumbar spine, you have to use many postural and muscular compensations to function causing pain to develop.

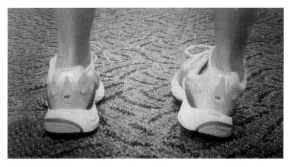

Some form of Valgus Wedging will help correct the over supination (on the right) from jamming the SI joint superiorly

Varus Wedges for Pronation does help pronators at times at the SI joint. This is usually discovered when you ask what symptoms are better after treatment. The mechanical function in pronators is simply to make the lower extremity more stable. It could be the correction of asymmetrical motion that has the biggest effect (one side pronating more than the other with asymmetrical treatment), or just the pure improvement in limb stability. It is important to remember that asymmetrical pronation causes a "functional short leg syndrome". Pronation allows the anterior pelvis to drop lower on the more pronated side, with asymmetrical symptoms caused by this pelvic tilt. I tend to use ¼ to ⅜ inch varus wedges with a greater amount when there is noticeable asymmetry on the more pronated side. I can then build this asymmetry into any orthotic device I design. The higher up the chain from the foot, the more these asymmetries seem to matter like ⅛ inch short leg or 2 degrees more varus tilt on one side.

Self Reduction Exercises are recommended when symptoms and pelvic unevenness are noted in supine testing mentioned above, or when checking for limb length discrepancy standing. There mechanical function is to make sure that the SI joint is in its centered position. I typically have the patient do a "bridge" in the office and check if the asymmetry or unevenness at least partially reduces. This becomes their home program at least once a day, and when symptoms arise. I try to see also if walking backwards 10 steps helps also, but to date I am less secure with that activity. Yet, it is easier to do midday than finding a place to lie down to perform the bridge exercise.

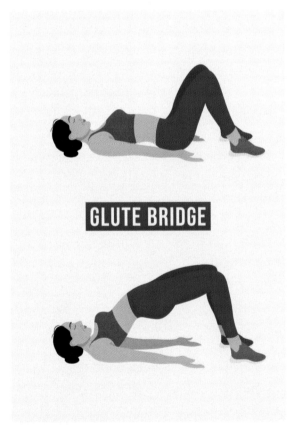

A Bridge or Glute Bridge is done once with a 5 second count going up and then down to self reduce a "stuck pelvis"

Shoe Changes would naturally occur if the goal is for better pronation support or supination support. However, I have found the sacro-iliac stress caused by heel strike in both a zero drop shoe (which puts an extension force at the knee), or too clunky a heeled shoe (driving ground reaction force up the leg). Also, the shoes themselves should be stable, not helping with the overall instability and wobble of the lower extremity. After I solve the pronation or supination issue, I typically like my patients to alternate shoes for a while until they are convinced one shoe is better for them or not. Make your patients tell you if they feel better in a heeled shoe, or a flat shoe, to start them thinking about the biomechanics.

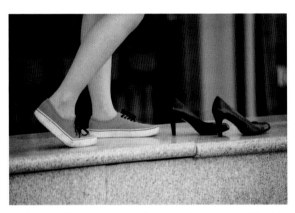

What makes your patient feel better with SI or Low Back Pain?

Practical Biomechanics Question #413: Patients that you are treating biomechanically will have back pain/SI joint pain. What 4 mechanical changes were discussed in the preceding section may help? Answer: 698

Lower Back Pain

The story of Maurice has to be told in a book on biomechanics for podiatrists. It of course is a success story, and in many ways a sad reflection on how the medical world is spinning. Maurice was a scholarship golfer when in his freshman year of college came down with terrible back pain which sidelined him from golf. For 2 years, the doctors and physical therapists and trainers, could only give him temporary help, and he could not play a single hole in golf. He was so desperate that he flew to Las Vegas for some micro surgery, which also proved unsuccessful. So, he then started a two year 3 times a week relationship with chiropractic, but again only got several hours at a time of temporary relief. In desperation, the chiropractor on the last visit looked down at his feet on the table, and referred to me because of his flat feet.

When I met Maurice, he was sitting and I heard his story. I then watched him walk and he was dominant to his right side. Dominance means that he put more weight on that side. It is one of the clues that a short leg may be present, but of course can be from muscle spasms, pelvic tilts, and scoliosis. Doing a cursory limb length examination, it revealed about ½ inch difference with his left leg being shorter. Due to the 4 year duration, he was now in graduate school, I decided to get an AP Pelvic Standing X Ray barefoot in a normal stance with knees straight to be positive what the exact measurement was. It turned out he was 22 mm or around 7/8th inch short on his right side. You can only imagine what this caused during a golf swing.

During the next 2 weeks all his shoes were built up to 7/8th inch, and within a month played 10 full rounds of golf in 12 days in Palm Desert, California. Yes, I am proud, but the key was simply in the gait evaluation. Maurice went off his merry way, I never did make him orthotic devices for his flatfeet. I didn't really have to at this stage. What I will never forget, well before we knew his treatment was a success, when I watched him walk he commented that I was the only one to watch him walk in the preceding four years. Astounding since it is the answer to so many problems.

Besides limb length discrepancies as the cause of low back pain, Dr. Howard Dananberg popularized the theory of "Sagittal Plane Facilitation." The root of the theory is that low back pain can occur when the forward motion of the foot is blocked, jarring the low back. He felt control at the rear part of the foot was useless, that motion at the forefoot was key. He partnered with Brooks Shoe Company to make their kinetic wedge to allow the big toe joint to move better. I have incorporated, or at least always acknowledged, that the design of the foot orthotic or shoe should never block this forward (sagittal plane) motion. Allowing the first metatarsal to plantar flex is a vital component to my Inverted Orthotic Technique.

Both the stabilization of excessive pronation or excessive supination have been implied in treatment for low back pain by lower extremity biomechanists. Excessive supination has always been a low back killer and I do my best eliminating that motion (which could be inherent to the foot or just particular shoes worn at times).

I have to mention that the timing of mechanical support, including shoe changes, may have to wait for the acute nature of the problem to calm down. Fortunately, I am typically called into consultation with these patients when their problem is chronic back pain, sometimes after a surgery or two which was only partially successful or rarely unsuccessful.

To tie this into Chapter 3 and 4 on gait and biomechanical examination, with low back pain the most important examinations to do in 10 minutes (or 20 minutes) are:
- Limb Length Discrepancy Evaluation
- Gait Signs or LLD, Excessive Pronation, or Excessive Supination
- Tight Hamstrings

Common Mechanical Changes with Low Back Pain (with the common ones used in RED)
1. Lifts for limb length discrepancy
2. Varus Wedging
3. Neural Flossing
4. Valgus Wedging
5. Custom Orthotic Devices
6. Hamstring Stretches
7. Shoe Changes
8. Shoe Modifications
9. Shock Absorbing Insoles
10. Sciatic Nerve Protection
11. Training Modifications

Lifts for limb length discrepancy is vital to my practice and I get MD referrals for leg length discrepancies all the time. Their mechanical function is to level the spine eliminating compensations and neural tension symptoms. I will refer you to my upcoming chapter on Limb Length Discrepancy for the subtleties, or golden rules, of correcting for a short leg. However, gait should clue you in to a possible short leg, and taking AP Pelvic Standing X Rays in normal stance barefoot may be crucial based on relative importance of being exact or the difficulty of finding good landmarks. The mantra used in limb length correction is "Start Low and Go Slow".

Practical Biomechanics Question #414: What are the 5 main gait signs that someone may have a short leg causing lower back pain? Answer: 698

Practical Biomechanics Question #415: Theorize the pros and cons of using a heel lift as your only treatment for leg length discrepancy. Answer: 698

Practical Biomechanics Question #416: If the mantra for treating Short Leg Syndrome is "Start Low and Go Slow" why did Maurice in the preceding story have ⅞ inch lifts placed on all his shoes immediately?

Varus Wedging is the first and sometimes the only treatment you will need as a podiatrist for low back pain when your gait evaluation finds excessive pronation as a possible cause. The mechanical functions are many and will be discussed here: reduce unsteadiness, eliminate asymmetries of function, allow for Sagittal Plane Facilitation, and decrease neural tension at the tarsal tunnel and piriformis. Pronation produces terrible unsteadiness in gait and pronation support can help ease the protective tension that develops at the low back. This seems to be a common compensation for foot instability to make your trunk and upper extremities stiff. The stiffer the back in gait, the more the stress of walking collects there. Also, excessive pronation can be the tipping point for a nervous system on edge. The sciatic nerve is irritated by the pronation motion particularly at the tarsal tunnel and piriformis. This increased neural tension can cause increased symptoms in the foot and in the low back. The wedges are typically ¼ to ⅜ inch and should be on both sides unless you are also treating a short leg. However, it is really important for the patient to differentiate these separate treatments right from the start. How does the patient feel with lifts, or how does the patient feel with pronation control? Also, asymmetrical pronation, which should be treated with more pronation control on the more pronated side, causes a functional short leg syndrome with all its symptoms. We also know that excessive pronation, with its dorsally jamming of the first metatarsal, can cause a blocking of propulsion and a jarring of the low back at heel lift.

Practical Biomechanics Question #417: When we measure (by many methods) that one foot pronates twice as much as the other side, which foot is acting as the short leg?

Practical Biomechanics Question #418: How does excessive pronation cause an apropulsive gait in some patients? How does that apropulsive gait potentially cause low back pain? Answer: 698

Neural Flossing is a common physical therapy treatment with low back pain. Its mechanical function is to eliminate or reduce neural tension in the lower extremity. I have had so many patients with low back pain that were started with neural flossing or gliding that symptoms they thought were musculoskeletal were reduced. One patient in particular had years of bouts of plantar fasciitis and the neural flossing kept these symptoms at a minimum. The problem therefore was probably plantar heel nerve entrapment (Baxter's).

Valgus Wedging is crucial in the supinators with low back pain. Their mechanical function is to allow heel contact pronation when the whole lower extremity is internally rotating. These are typically ⅛ to ¼ inch. Whereas a little pronation is normal and healthy for lower extremity motion, a little contact phase supination is terrible. Therefore, I do whatever it takes to remove it from the patient's biomechanics. Shoes are a big cause and I encourage you to have the patients walk with and without their shoes, and also bring for a visit a selection of their common shoe gear. Patients may only be supinators when they put shoes on their feet. In chapter 5 of Book 2, I discussed the simple to complex treatments for supination. Contact phase supination jars the back and SI joints and has to be mitigated.

Practical Biomechanics Question #418: What does it mean to have both medial and lateral instability? How could that affect your treatment for low back pain? A: 698

Custom Orthotic Devices are the big guns biomechanical control of the lower extremity control. They can let you do a better job controlling pronation or supination forces. The chapter on custom orthotic devices upcoming in Book 4 goes over the various orthotic devices for increasing pronation or supination support. And, as I said before, some pronation is normally fine, but please attempt to remove all contact phase supination found. I also want to advise against the practice of applying lifts to orthoses. Keep them separate, at least until you have worked out the role of each in your treatment. This is especially true when patients have increased back or knee pain with your inserts and it can be hard to tell if the problem is the lift or the orthotic device. The other type of custom orthotic device occasionally used for low back pain is the Hannaford, or a similar device. These are devices, and labs have quite a few choices, that combine stability with an important cushion to dampen the shock wave going up the leg.

Practical Biomechanics Question #419: What parts of a standard custom made functional foot orthotic device could cause low back pain and why? Answer: 698

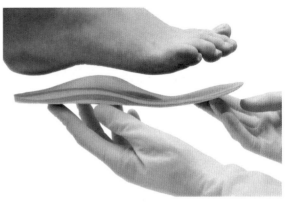

It is good to know the common causes of low back pain produced by custom orthotic devices so that proper adjustments can be made

Hamstring Stretches is the classic lower extremity treatment for low back pain. We all know that the hamstrings when tight pull downward on the ischial tuberosities (our sit bones) and straighten the normally curved lumbar spine producing disc compressions. Also, this effect on the spine causes many muscles to tighten to protect the spine, or to shift the center of gravity forward too much. It is important to stretch the upper and lower hamstrings separately as has been previously outlined.

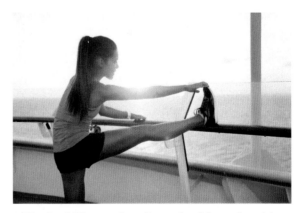

Typical Hamstring Stretch although with low back pain I de-emphasize the toe touch part and make sure the level you are at is stable

Practical Biomechanics Question #420: What are the two main types of Hamstring Stretches, and which one is demonstrated in the photo above? Answer: 699

Shoe Changes are primarily for better shock absorption which typically help low back pain sufferers. The heel height will always be a debate for low back pain, but I have found 50% of my back patients love most heels, and 50% need flats only. I am sure it has something to do with the curve of their spine as the lordotic curve increases the higher the heel. Perhaps, my flat backed patients love heels, and my more lordotic patients hate heels. Shoe changes can also be needed to get more depth to house our lifts, wedges, or orthotic devices. Shoe changes can be needed to help the varus or valgus support, or heel height changes (15 mm to zero drop range on the market). Your low back sufferers may have already decided the best type of shoe for them and it is crucial to know in your biomechanical assessment.

Shoe Modifications for low back pain are typically adding midsole or outsole varus or valgus wedging, or lifts for the short leg. So many of my patients with back pain wear very unsupportive shoes for long hours at a time, so a good relationship with a local cobble skilled at adding wedges or lifts to shoes is very important. At times, flat shoes can have heels added, or heels removed, but the cobbler needs to see the shoes beforehand to decide which ones that they can work with.

Shock Absorbing Insoles to help with the reduction of the ground reactive force traveling up the leg. I love both Spenco and Poron materials, or one of their knockoffs, for pure shock absorption. At times, a simple heel cushion is enough, with the least shoe crowding potential. But, at times a heel pad of any type increases the force up the leg, or adds to instability by lifting the patient out of the shoe, or produces a clunkiness in gait as the weight goes forward. In most of these instances, a full length insert (some cut out at the sulcus to give the toes some room), is the ideal way of these insoles. And, you should always watch the patient walk after any adjustment to check on stability and get the patient's feedback. Always err on making them more stable with what you do.

Sciatic Nerve Protection for low back pain is just a smart thing to do. The patients need to know what stresses the sciatic nerve since it may be involved to some extent (like bending your knee when you lift, the appropriate method of getting up and down from lying, and why bending over is bad from the waist). I prefer a physical therapist to instruct my patients on this, but I seem to always want to add my 2 cents.

Training Modifications really depend on the nature of the problem. Twisting and the impact of running are avoided at the start. Walking, swimming, recumbent bikes, and ellipticals are normally the first aspects of physical training after an acute injury. Since most of my patients are chronic low back sufferers, it is important to get a history of what they are doing exercise wise

that causes low back pain and see if there
are any workarounds that you can devise.

Chapter 8: Biomechanical Concepts

(by Carlos Martinez Sebastian and Alvaro Gomez Carrion)

The following is an important discussion of fantastic observations made by incredible individuals in the field of lower extremity biomechanics. Where individual practitioners may find their clinical practices focused more on one approach over others presented by these various concepts, it is the purpose of this book to present them as all contributing to the body of knowledge we call lower extremity biomechanics. These concepts are not mutually exclusive. Dr Blake in his practice uses all of these observations or theories to help his patients. It is therefore vitally important to understand the concepts presented to fully treat or at least understand the dynamics at play in designing rehabilitation protocols, designing foot inserts, planning surgical procedures, and helping pain syndromes in general. As emphasized in Chapters 1 and 2 of this Book series, treating the mechanics of a patient may vary from visit to visit, as you treat the individual patient.

The authors encourage all those interested in lower extremity biomechanics to discover the benefits of a kinetic wedge, invert a patient 25 degrees, add a medial and lateral Kirby skive, evaluate where the center of pressure is, find subtalar joint neutral in a patient with bowlegs, and observe which plane is dominant in a severe pronator. These are just some of the more common examples of how these concepts work together, and will help your practice of lower extremity biomechanics.

Root Concepts

This way of observing the foot and the lower extremity has as its main author Dr. Merton L. Root. He was considered the father of podiatric biomechanics and is the first to lay the foundations on which all current biomechanics will be developed; along with orthotic therapy. He presents some biophysical criteria of normality that are the following: verticality of the tibia, vertical calcaneal position, neutral position of the subtalar, locking of the midtarsal joint in maximum pronation to achieve the forefoot-hindfoot relationship in the same working plane, 2nd to 4th dorsi-flexed metatarsals, and 1st and 5th metatarsals in the same working plane (the last 2 points creating the metatarsal arch from medial to lateral).

Practical Biomechanics Question #421: With Dr Root and colleagues, they were trying to establish a reference point for biomechanics and subsequent treatment in their classifications of normalcy and deformity. "Normal" was really "Ideal" so that there would be no deformities causing pathology. How did they attempt to measure a forefoot to rearfoot deformity? A: 699

When deviations from these criteria of normality occur, there would be compensations made by the body for these variations in structure or other soft tissue problems. These compensations are classified according to the deformity, for example, the supinated forefoot would produce a compensation for a valgus hindfoot. There are varus and valgus hindfoot deformities, and varus and valgus forefoot deformities. Through the plantar supports (called functional foot orthotic devices), we can correct these compensations by supporting the deformities, and thus improve the pathology.

Practical Biomechanics Question #422: If the deformity is a high degree of Tibial Varum, what would the normal compensation be at the foot? Answer: 699

Practical Biomechanics Question #423: If the deformity is a first metatarsal too high (metatarsus primus elevatus), what would the compensation be at the rear foot? (699)

These concepts are based on the functioning of the foot correctly when the subtalar joint is in or near neutral position, together with the functioning of two axes of the midtarsal joint. The longitudinal axis and the oblique axis would provide the transition of movement between the hindfoot and the forefoot (typically stiffening with subtalar supination and becoming hypermobile with subtalar pronation). Following these established criteria of normality, the goal of orthotic therapy is to eliminate foot compensations (by supporting the deformities found) and bring it to the neutral position and be able to meet the criteria. For this, the taking of plaster casts prioritizes the neutral position of the AST (subtalar joint), the midtarsal joints in maximum pronation and the

forefoot-hindfoot relationship preserved in the same plane (only when there is no forefoot deformity present).

Practical Biomechanics Question #424: When a neutral suspension cast is taken (in subtalar neutral and midtarsal joints maximally pronated), what are the 3 types of forefoot alignments found? A: 699

Practical Biomechanics Question #425: Dr Root taught balancing frontal plane deformities by taking a good impression cast was key to many foot problems. What could a tight achilles or weak posterior tibial tendon cause to complicate the stability Dr Root was seeking? A: 699

Sagittal plane facilitation

The sagittal plane facilitation concept was described by Podiatrist Howard J. Dananberg in his first article in 1986. Those of us in lower extremity biomechanics owe Dr Dananberg for emphasizing sagittal plane evaluation and the relationship of the foot to the back (among other great knowledge shared). The author describes that human locomotion occurs thanks to the rocking phase, where the lower limb that is not supporting the weight of the body (swing phase in open kinetic chain) is able to move forward without resistance to friction. When performing this previous movement, the body's center of mass moves forward creating a lever arm on which the body will pivot just following heel contact and forefoot loading. The other foot is on the floor receiving the full weight of the body and carrying it through it. The ability to support the weight of the body is thanks to the synergy of all the joints of the lower limb, the stability of the back, hip, knee, ankle and of course the foot.

The foot that is in a closed kinetic chain has the mechanical ability to transfer body weight through its structure. In the contact phase it occurs through the first rocker, where the rounded shape of the heel allows the reception of body weight to be transferred forward. In the middle stance phase the second rocker is produced with the ankle joint allowing the tibia to move forward to transfer the load to the forefoot. It takes about 10 degrees of dorsiflexion to avoid blockage of this motion at the ankle. The author cites the importance of the take-off phase, because it is when the foot, in a closed kinetic chain, transfers the body weight to the other foot, that the swing phase begins. This lever fulcrum allows the entire weight of the body to be transferred thanks to the capacity of the metatarsophalangeal joints (the third rocker), especially from the first metatarsophalangeal joint. The function of the plantar fascia, described by Hicks more than 50 years ago, reveals the ability of the foot to supinate in the take-off phase through the Windlass mechanism. This mechanism consists in that the first metatarsophalangeal joint performs a dorsal flexion in the take-off phase, in which the fascia rolls up like the mechanism of a windlass, generating a tension movement in the fascia and supination occurs. The tension in the fascia generates the blockage of the calcaneocuboid joint creating a stability between the hindfoot and the midfoot. This maneuver provides the foot

with the function of being a rigid lever during propulsion. Approximate 65 degree dorsiflexion is required to allow proper limb lift-off.

Practical Biomechanics Question #426: What are the 3 rockers of the foot allowing smooth forward motion during the stance phase of gait? Answer: 699

If during the take-off phase, the longitudinal axis of the metatarsal is parallel to the ground (in a very pronated foot so no plantar declination of the first metatarsal), the foot will not have an efficient capacity to transfer body weight. On the other hand, when the longitudinal axis of the metatarsal is plantigrade to the ground (more vertical) and the first metatarsal performs the correct plantar flexion, the foot will have greater capacity and efficiency in transferring body weight to the other lower limb. When we find alterations in the transfer of energy through the lower limb, we may find a foot free of pain, but we can find involvement of other proximal structures such as the knee, hip and lower back in pain patterns. This implies that the foot will not complain, but the rest of the leg to low back may complain.

This is a great time to remember the mantra of gait evaluation: Heel lift of one side should occur just prior to heel contact of the other side.

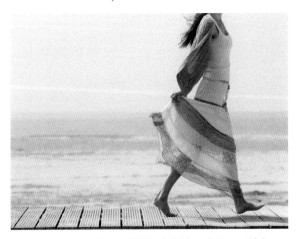

Perfect Timing of Heel Lift of One Side occurring before Heel Contact of the Other Side in Normal Propulsive Gait (Best seen from the Side View of the Sagittal Plane)

Functional hallux limitus is described as the etiology where the proximal phalanx loses the ability to move in dorsiflexion on the metatarsal head during walking. This pathology can be overlooked on examination, since most present a good range of motion in the joint non weight bearing, and this is observed and measured in weight bearing. The duration of this blockage or inability to perform dorsiflexion during ambulation occurs for about 100 milliseconds, being almost imperceptible to the human eye. This block would be precursor to Hallux Rigidus, where micro traumas produced in the joint would cause degeneration of it. Improper function of this joint will cause the delay or blocking of heel lift, generating compensations in other joints having the ability to move in the sagittal plane, as occurs in the midtarsal joint with arch pain developing.

Practical Biomechanics Question #427: If functional hallux limitus can be the

precursor to degenerative changes in the big toe joint, what advice should you give all your patients who present with functional hallux limitus? Answer: 700

The Synergy of Flexing dorsally during the third rocker is vital so that the rest of the joints proximal can carry out their function in the right way. The analogy represented by a scissor lift or jack, where the hip, knee, ankle and foot extend and flex in opposite directions. A failure in a joint would mean the affectation of the rest and movement of the sagittal plane could not occur.

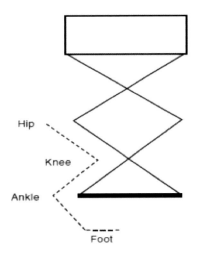

Copied with Permission of Author showing as One Joint Flexes Another Extends in the Lower Extremity (Big Toe Joint Flexes, Ankle Extends, Knee Flexes, Hip Extends) as the foot readies itself for Take-off

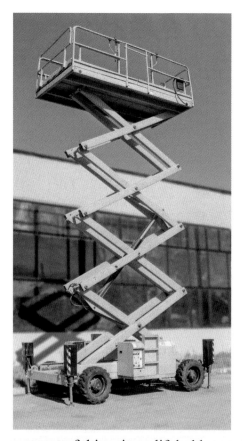

The concept of this scissor lift holds true for the body. When one joint flexes in gait, the next one in line will extend, and this occurs up and down the lower extremity chain.

With the development of technology, we have been able to verify how the blockade affects the sagittal plane and the plantar pressures during the walking. When there is a blockage, the energy stored needs to be dissipated or transferred, that is why the following 5 plane offsets (compensations) commonly occur in the sagittal plane.

1) Alteration of the takeoff of the heel: There is a delay in heel lift or heel lift block, which generates pronation through the midtarsal in the second half of the phase midstance support. This can be related to a weak achilles tendon.

2) Toes raise in phase takeoff: it's a continuation of the first compensation, when the heel does not take off in the final phase, there is a slow and apropulsive gait, does not have the ability to efficiently transfer the body weight to the other member/foot in the swing phase. Again, could be related to a weak achilles tendon.

3) Reverse Step: When you are blocked at the first metatarsophalangeal joint, the foot generates a supination moment and transfers weight to the external/lateral column, which is easily visible with loading of the lesser metatarsals with the pressure platform. These feet can present in static examination with a rearfoot valgus deformity (which tends to stay pronated in propulsion), but in dynamics will supinate to avoid blockage.

4) Adduction or Abduction in phase take-off: Because the body weight should flow through the foot, the compensatory mechanisms may generate internal rotation at the hip with an adducted forefoot to prevent the block of the first metatarsophalangeal joint (in toe the gait), and equally as well generate external rotation (out toe the gait) and then they roll over the medial part of the forefoot.

5) Knee and Low Back compensation of the body: When a block of this sagittal plane flow occurs, the knee can't flex forward in the phase of take off, generating a possible compensation in bending the lumbar spine forward instead.

Practical Biomechanics Question #428: What are the 5 common compensations that individuals will take when they have difficulty bending their big toe joint at the start of the propulsive phase of gait? (700)

Once the pathology of the functional hallux limitus is recognized, we can design our plantar orthosis in order to facilitate movement in the sagittal plane. The Kinetic Wedge® consists of a piece designed to facilitate plantar flexion of the first metatarsal and dorsiflexion of the proximal phalanx during the takeoff phase. This piece functions to eliminate the resistance to dorsal bending under head of first metatarsal by giving support to the rest of metatarsal heads, and first toe, with a material of a soft density. The gap can be filled with material of a density less than rest. The proximal bevel of the hole is parallel to the axis of the first metatarsal, and the distal bevel parallel to the line of gait progression. Most orthotic labs have their version.

Practical Biomechanics Question #429: What is the number one treatment for functional Hallux limitus? Answer: 700

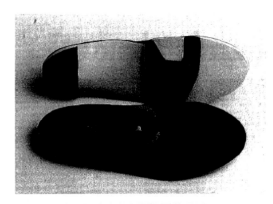

Kinetic Wedge ® demonstrated
Permission given by the Author

Locally, the Kinetic Wedge® has the ability to increase the declination of the first metatarsal performing plantar flexion of this, and of the reduction of the prime adduction movement of the first metatarsal in the transverse plane. The effect of sagittal plane facilitation with plantar supports is described in the scientific literature with big results. Subjects were collected with postural pain in the back, knee joint, and temporomandibular, and after the use of the plantar supports 77% obtained an improvement of their symptoms between 50% and 100%. And the other 23% got an improvement between 25% and 50%. All continued to use their templates and they did not stop using them.

In another study, 32 subjects were dispensed plantar supports who had pathology in the lumbar area. Their pain scale was evaluated for the impact of pain on your daily life via The Quebec Back Pain Disability Scale. It was found that after use of plantar supports pain relief was obtained lower back symptomatology.

Practical Biomechanics Question #430: The movement from our heel at foot strike to the end of push off should be smooth. Any block in that motion will give problems somewhere in the body. When in gait does the low back get the most stressed according to the Sagittal Facilitation Theory? Answer: 700

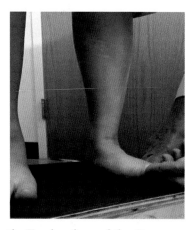

Static Evaluation of the Presence of Functional Hallux Limitus in pronated foot position (Chapter 4)

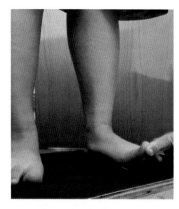

Static Evaluation reveals no Functional Hallux Limitus while the Patient is standing on a supportive Custom Orthotic Device

Midtarsal Joint Function

The midtarsal joint is an important structure in the function of the foot, and is the transition between the hindfoot and the forefoot. It is made up of two joints, the talus-navicular and the calcaneocuboid.

The midtarsal joint was described as a joint with two joint axes of movement. This concept has been taught in the last thirty years, without scientific evidence of its validation.

Manter in 1940 carried out a study of both the subtalar joint as well as the midtarsal joint, and emphasizes the importance of both in foot functionality. He proposes the concept that the midtarsal joint has two axes of movements. The long axis would be located at 15 degrees to the transverse plane, and 9 degrees to the sagittal plane. The oblique axis would be located 57 degrees relative to the sagittal plane and 52 degrees relative to the transverse plane. The Longitudinal axis mainly provided the inversion and eversion movement; and the oblique axis provided the movements of dorsiflexion-abduction and plantarflexion-adduction. Related to the pathologies of the foot, the author described the oblique axis motion related with flat feet and arch loss associated with the pronation movement.

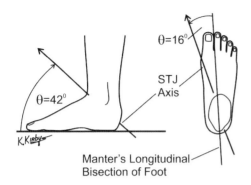

θ=16°

STJ Axis

θ=42°

K.Kirby

Manter's Longitudinal Bisection of Foot

Photo Courtesy of Dr Kevin Kirby
Showing the proposed subtalar joint axis
deviated in the sagittal and transverse
planes

Practical Biomechanics Question #431:
Manter's classic work laid the foundation
80 years ago of the midtarsal joint having
many axes. How many did he believe
existed and what were their names? A:700

Van Langelaan's groundbreaking study used
the technique of X-ray photometry for the
study of ten feet of cadavers. They
implanted small metallic marks, about 2
mm in diameter, in the tibia, fibula,
calcaneus, talus, navicular, and cuboid of
each cadaver. This allowed them to know
the accurate locations during
three-dimensional views of each of these
bones, the external rotation movement, and
inside of the leg under load on a platform.
With these locations in space of the bones
of the midtarsal region now known in each
step, rotational movement and
three-dimensional translation of the tarsal
bones could be calculated for a step. From
this information, the axes could be known
as spirals of the movement of a
bone relative to another. This study

showed that the axes of the foot do not
behave as hinge-type axes, but as helical
axes; that is, axes that have
rotational movements and translation
depending on the position of the
foot.

Practical Biomechanics Question #432: The
Van Langelaan study showed that the axes of
foot joints were of what type? A: 700

Nester in his studies of the midtarsal joint
highlights that the physical principles of
kinematics will not allow a rigid body
(bone) to move in opposite directions, as
proposed by the model of the two axes. That
is to say, that the pronated midtarsal joint
around its oblique axis cannot also supinate
around its longitudinal axis. The objective
of the study was to evaluate the relationship
of scaphoid and cuboid with the calcaneus
during in-plane leg transverse movements,
through a system of 3D motion recording.
His team arrived at the conclusion that there
is only one axis that allows movement in all
three coordinate planes. The measures
were carried out under load, respecting
the kinematic function of ligaments and
muscles. They got a 37.9 axis degrees
relative to the transverse plane and 29
degrees from the sagittal plane.

Practical Biomechanics Question #433:
Christopher Nester concluded that the
midtarsal joint only has one axis that moves
in all three body planes. By removing the
concept of a longitudinal axis of the
midtarsal joint, how does a forefoot
supinatus or pronatus develop? A: 700

Nester, in his previous articles, describes a transition to a new biomechanical model of the midtarsal joint in which a single axis is able to describe all movements of this joint. The new coordinate model proposed by the author incorporates calcaneus as a local reference point that allows it to maintain the same clinical terminology that was described for the previous model of the two axes. It's not changing much our clinical model of midtarsal joint function, but is clearing up this scientific character that allows us clearly establish a link between clinical models and models of joint experiments. The above terminology allows you explain a supination movement around the longitudinal axis and pronation around the oblique axis, and new proposal that replaces the above would be: a movement of inversion on the X axis, dorsiflexion on the Z axis, and abduction on the Y axis. We can assume that the joints such as the midtarsal, scapho-cuneal and cuneo-metatarsal have great relevance in foot functionality. Nester studied and described the motion for each foot bone during walking on feet cadaverous, finding conclusions of vital importance for the clinic practice. Based on the average data of movement between the scaphoid and talus, cuneiform and scaphoid, and first cuneiform and first metatarsal, group a total of 29, the axis was 21 degrees in the sagittal plane. These data were compared with the combination of movement of the ankle joint and the subtalar joint, which produced a total of 28, or 81° in the sagittal plane. When we compare the set of joints we found that both are capable of reproducing almost similar motion kinematics, the clinical importance of midtarsal, scaphocuneal and cuneo-metatarsal, are in the same scale of value that gave it to the subtalar joint and talar ankle joint.

Practical Biomechanics Question #434: Whereas the exact measurements are a bit confusing here, needless to say, the one axis of the midtarsal joint theory makes sense. What are the 4 main joints below the knee which help in forward motion? A: 700

It has also been shown that there is coordination in the pattern of movement of the ankle joint and hip joint to the midtarsal joint in the sagittal plane during the takeoff phase, highlighting the role of shortening of the arc in the propulsion phase. After various investigations, it was the conclusion that, the midtarsal would have the ability to move in all three planes of space, through a single axis, being able to have dominance at some level. This single axis would cover the whole or the sum of these three reference axes: the medial-lateral axis (allows motion in the sagittal plane), the vertical axis (allows motion in the transverse plane), and the anterior–posterior axis (allows motion in the frontal or coronal plane).

Practical Biomechanics Question #435: Foot joints have axes that allow motion in all three cardinal planes, and thus called triplanar. Axes that are more vertical allow a greater amount of what type of motion?

Tissue Stress

An external force applied to an object

will cause strain and/or deformity. Tension is the ability of a material to develop internal resistance to forces exerted against it. The deformity is the amount of deformity suffered by a material when subjected to a force. Depending on the nature of the external force that acts on it, a structure can develop stress as compression, traction, and/or shearing.

Practical Biomechanics Question #436: What are the 3 types of stress that can cause injury to our patients? Answer: 701

The axial force can occur in either of two ways: compression and traction. A structure is defined to be under compression if the axial force tends to shorten it. If the axial force causes a structure to elongate, then it is said to be under traction. Another form of force on a structure is called shearing, which occurs when there is a horizontal shift of one layer over another of the same structure.

In 1995, McPoil and Hunt promoted the idea that mechanical foot therapy should be directed towards resolution of tissue tension in what they called "the stress model of fabrics". The tissue stress proposition is based on the concept of that when any of the structural components of the foot or lower extremity is situated under more stress than they can bear by location, type, and magnitude, the structural component can be ultimately damaged, which can lead to pain at the site damaged or injured.

Practical Biomechanics Question #437: McPoil and Hunt really changed how some people felt we should be treating patients. Whereas orthotic devices described by Root and Dananberg work well with this concept, the emphasis of Tissue Stress is on what treatment modalities? Answer: 701

In engineering, the method of relationship between the force applied to a material and the deformation is represented by a stress-strain diagram. This method graph will help us understand the material properties of organic and inorganic nature. In it they analyze the pathomechanics of overuse injuries, utilizing a load-strain curve that consists of two zones: an elastic region and a plastic region, delimited by the microfault zone. This diagram shows whether the material is ductile or rigid, and also at what level of tension changes from being elastic to plastic. Inside the elastic (linear) region we will have the origin, where there is no load, and the endpoint called the elastic limit, where we find the limit of that linear gradual increase of load without reaching the loss of elasticity. In the plastic region occurs a stress applied to the material beyond its elastic limit causing a permanent deformation of the material. The further increase in load leads the material to its ultimate capacity stress, when failures begin to occur, leading to fracture or rupture of that structure in question.

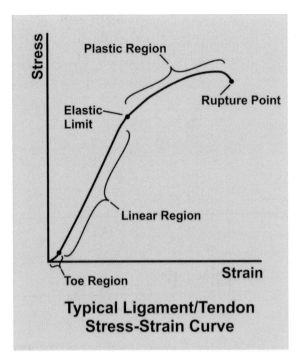

Typical Ligament/Tendon Stress-Strain Curve

This image is courtesy of Dr Kevin Kirby to explain the Tissue Stress concept

Practical Biomechanics Question #438: The plastic region to the rupture point can be applied to tendons, bones, and ligaments. What structure when damaged can have the most long lasting and devastating problems?

With respect to the lower limbs, weight bearing activities such as standing, walking, jogging, or running for a period of time occurs with constant stress on the tissues, which depending on the load, can be found in the region of elastic deformation where there is no tissue damage. Conversely, increased load due to a biomechanical problem such as pronation, can result in a deformation in the tissues beyond the microfault zone (elastic limit), reaching the plastic region. This load increase in tissues for long periods of time and excessive use produces damage resulting in injury. The goal of the clinician using proposed tissue stress, to the biomechanical therapy, is to reduce the stress in the structural component of a foot and/or lower extremity injury so that it works according to its rank of elasticity. In the case of a structure that was damaged significantly or weakened, the stresses need to be further reduced, in order to allow the optimal tissue healing.

The first step is to identify the anatomical structure that is the source of the patient's complaint. The clinician must have a detailed appreciation of the anatomy of the foot and lower extremity, including surface signals of anatomical structures that are not easily palpable, but can be discovered through specific testing, to determine the exact identity of the structure of pain. These tests must include pain production assessment by manual pressure on the specific anatomical structures, during muscle resistance activity, and/or during the range of passive movement of the joints. There will also be necessary diagnostic tests, such as ultrasound radiography, and sometimes invasive in such as diagnosis by anesthesia.

Practical Biomechanics Question #439: Chapter 2 in Book 1 discusses the thought process of when to image, how to keep pain between 0-2, etc. Many injuries, like ankle tendonitis syndrome, have superficial pain when the problem is really deep. Explain the concept of when a superficial complaint is not getting better why you should think "deep". Answer: 701

The second step is to determine structural and/or functional variables that may be the source of the pathological forces of the damaged structure. Clinical data derived from the biomechanical examination of the foot and lower extremity such as, muscle testing, range of motion examinations, and gait assessment, are parts of our comprehensive understanding of how pathological forces can be generated to cause damage to the individual. Also, creating a model of the functional and structural variables that may be affecting stress in a structure will give an idea of how the external loads can be altered to reduce stress on a structure. These models can be simple or complex, but exact enough to predict how the methods of clinical treatment may mechanically affect the stresses in a specific anatomical structure.

Practical Biomechanics Question #440: Chapter 1 of Book 1 (and then later in Chapter 2) discusses the Rule of 3 which helps in our model of how an injury occurs and how we can treat that injury. Discuss a possible Rule of 3 for big toe joint pain (many examples exist). Answer: 701

The third step in a treatment plan, both mechanical and therapeutic, should be formulated, and will be more effective if to achieve the following objectives in the treatment for each patient: 1-) reduce pathological load forces in structural components damaged, 2-) optimize the entire step function, and 3-) prevent any other pathology or symptoms to

occur. The proper use of tissue tension approach allows the clinician to treat foot pathologies and more difficult lower extremity conditions mechanically.

The clinician must have a firm foundation of interpretation as to the many mechanical variables that can both increase to decrease internal forces that act in that structure during activities such as walking and running, and injury mechanisms concerning every sport. Mechanical treatment techniques; such as elongation and consolidation of muscles, heel cups, plantar supports, recommendations in the shoe design and orthopedic gadgets; can be evaluated and established, in an attempt to reduce stress and reduce pain.

Practical Biomechanics Question #441: The tissue stress concept typically uses many modalities to help reduce stress. What would 5 modalities commonly used to reduce stress in an injured posterior tibial tendon? Answer: 701

Practical Biomechanics Question #442: What 5 treatment modalities can be utilized to reduce stress in an achilles injury? (701)

Practical Biomechanics Question #443: What 5 treatment modalities commonly used to reduce stress on a big toe joint injury? Answer: 701

Physics Concepts

When the accelerations are zero, the net moment and force that act on the segments of the foot should also be at zero. To calculate the moment about any axis of a joint, the spatial location of the axis of the articulation, direction, magnitude, and the point of application of the forces, must be determined. The moment equals distance perpendicular from the line of action of force to the hinge axis. Every time we walk, we run, we jump or develop any movement of our bodies there are forces acting through the joints. These forces can come from an external source such as ground reaction force (FRS) that interacts with the foot, or may do it internally like muscle contraction or ligamentous tension. Whatever its origin, internal or external, that force will cause 2 other types of forces to act on the joint: the forces of rotation and compression. The ratio of rotational force and compression as a result of force acting through a joint axis, is determined by the angle at which the vector of that force is applied relative to the axis articulating with. The force vectors that act directly towards (parallel) the joint axis will resolve to 100% of compressive force and 0% rotation force. On the other hand, force vectors acting on a joint axis with one direction perpendicular to its moment arm will resolve to 0% force compression and 100% strength rotation.

Practical Biomechanics Question #444: Force applied perpendicular to a joint axis produces what percentage of compression forces, and what percentage of rotation forces? Answer: 702

When an object is in equilibrium, the net force and moment acting on it must be equal to zero, since Newton's second law states that the net force applied to an object is equal to the mass of the object times the acceleration of the object. When the acceleration is zero, as when the object is at rest, the net force acting on the object must be zero.

Practical Biomechanics Question #445: What are Newton's 3 Laws? Answer: 702

Practical Biomechanics Question #446: Explain the basis of a Free Body Diagram on the ankle joint axis. Answer: 702

A second important concept for the understanding free body diagram analysis is that of torques. When two forces are applied to an object, and those forces are directly opposite each other, acting on the same line of action, then these two forces of opposing opposition will only cause compression to the object. Anyway, when those forces are not directly opposite each other and act along different lines of action, a couple of forces are created.

Practical Biomechanics Question #447: What is the definition of a Couple of Forces? Answer: 702

A couple of force will create a moment which will tend to make the object rotate. The magnitude of the moment will be equal to the magnitude of force times distance between the lines of action of the two forces. In a couple of forces though, there must be a net moment acting on the object that tends to make it rotate, and there should be the existence of a net force acting on the object that tends to make it move. Hence it is important to realize that both internal and external forces act on the object, they will affect whether the object is moved or rotated, and will affect the magnitude and distribution of stresses internally that act within the object.

Practical Biomechanics Question #448: The coupling of forces acts in our complex world of biomechanics with every step. Imagine the pronatory forces which act on the subtalar joint coupled with the supinatory forces acting to resist this pronation. Describe the typical external forces created on a pronatory foot in podiatric biomechanics daily. A: 702

Rotational Balance

Practical Biomechanics Question #449: Define a moment in physics in one sentence

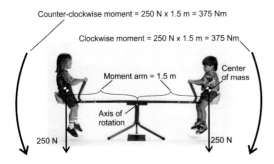

What is Rotational Equilibrium?

Photo Courtesy of Dr Kevin Kirby to illustrate Rotational Equilibrium with the use of a Seesaw

Dr Kevin Kirby said when the moments about a joint are equal to zero, we can say that the joint is in rotational equilibrium. This situation occurs when the sum of the

moments, as many pronatory as supinatory for instance, is equal to zero. For one foot to balance rotationally, the moments generated by the reactive forces of the ground must be counteracted by other anatomical structures. The action of muscles. such as the tibialis anterior, has the ability to generate supinatory moments around the axis of the subtalar joint, with other muscles producing pronatory moments. It is believed that the stress caused by unbalanced moments across a joint is the cause of many gait pathologies.

Practical Biomechanics Question #450: How would you explain how the subtalar joint is not in equilibrium when the heel is 14 degrees everted to the tibia bisection?

The net moment acting along the subtalar joint axis (AST) is a sum of all the moments of pronation and supination acting on any instant in time along the axis of the AST. The factors that can produce a moment in the axis of the AST are: GRF (Reaction Forces from the ground), forces acting through the ankle joint in the talus, muscular forces, forces of interosseous compression, and forces ligamentous extensible.

When GRF is equal to body weight, the net force acting on the body will be zero, and the body will be at rest, no acceleration vertical. The mechanical interaction of the GRF and body weight will help determine the magnitude of the forces (external load) acting on the foot during sports activities and weight. To keep the body erect and allow normal operation while standing, walking, running or doing other weight-bearing activities, there are internal forces present within the structural component of the foot and lower extremity and within the body memory. One of the forces most commonly recognized internally derives from the tensile forces that are generated by contractile activity muscle during weight bearing exercise. However, other internal forces, such as those derived from compressive forces that act within the bones of the body, and the tensile forces that act within the ligaments holding joints together, are as important as the others to allow correct posture and allow proper support of weight. Hence, both in the engineering, as in our experience daily with our patients, we understand that it is the combination of both external forces acting on an object and the internal forces that act within it, which determines how an object reacts mechanically to load forces that act on it. However, and very important, clinicians do not understand and appreciate so much that the magnitude of the internal forces acting on components of the foot and lower extremity structures is largely affected by the geometry, or anatomy, of the foot in relation to the loads that are applied. Understanding is both crucial and basic of how the relationship in the three dimensional components/structures of the foot are to the internal forces acting in those structures during weight bearing activities.

Practical Biomechanics Question #451: Clinicians considering the forces exerted on the body in sports will begin to adapt their treatment to minimize overload affects.

What are common treatment modalities that can help with this reduction of stress? 703

The axis localization technique at a joint in unloading is a pressure test modification of Dr. John Weed. His objective was to determine how far medial on the heel surface should be pushed to produce supination of the subtalar joint (AST). Dr Kevin Kirby modified this open kinetic chain technique applying prolonged pressure throughout the plantar aspect of the foot to see the response of the foot, while at the same time the thumb of the other hand is placed on the 4th and 5th head of the foot, detecting supination and pronation. In this test we find that the behavior of the foot may vary depending where we press on the plantar surface, and the "points of no rotation" will be marked on the sole coinciding with the axis of the AST. For this we will go along the sole, pressing the plantar surface, and causing supination when we exert pressure medial to the axis, and pronation when we exert pressure lateral to the axis. The point of no rotation corresponds to the location axis of the AST. It is important to understand both ground reaction force, and axis of the AST, since it will allow us to understand the type of lever arm needed to create a force to both correct pronation and supination.

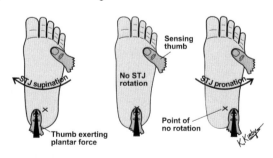

Illustration courtesy of Dr Kevin Kirby demonstrating the initial examination technique of finding the subtalar joint axis with typically 4 points of no rotation are found from proximal to distal

The clinician can learn where to put wedges or support especially in the medially and laterally deviated AST axis feet. For example, in the most lateral zone of the forefoot in a foot with a medially deviated axis will cause a greater moment of pronation through that axis. At the time of treatment this knowledge can guide us in the placement of wedges in the medial heel, where a foot with a severely deviated axis medially we will have less space to produce a moment of supination in a more standard orthosis..

Closed kinetic chain pronation (CCC) will cause the axis of the AST to internally rotate, plantarflex, and move medially; and the supination in CCC will cause that axis externally rotate, dorsiflex, and move laterally relative to the sole of the foot. A foot with a deviated AST axis medially will cause an increase of pronating moment arms, and a decrease in the arms supination when the FRS (ground reactive force) on the plantar structures of that foot. To the contrary, a foot with an axis of the AST deflected laterally will cause a increase in moment arms supination, and a decrease in pronator arms when the FRS on the plantar structures of that foot.

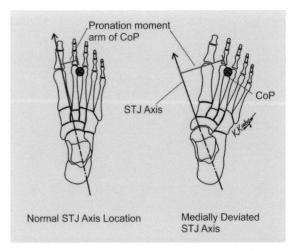

Photo Courtesy of Dr Kevin Kirby with the CoP representing all of the plantar surface pressure points (entire foot plantar pressure is pronatory around the subtalar joint axis when the axis is medially deviated)

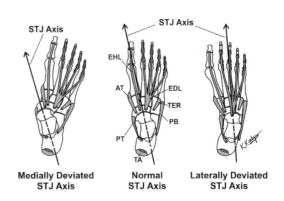

Photo Courtesy of Dr Kevin Kirby

After years analyzing the technique of AST palpation, Dr. Kevin Kirby observed that feet showing a normal gait function, the axis of the AST seen from the plantar surface is directed from the lateral aspect of the heel to the space of the first two heads of the metatarsals. The starting point is presented from the posterior plantar area of the calcaneus to a superior position-distal by passing through the neck of the talus.

In a normal foot with the axis of the AST slightly pronated from your neutral position, that axis will remain almost above the first head metatarsal and sesamoid (center). During pronation in CCC, the axis of AST internally rotates and translates medially in relation to the head of the metatarsal and sesamoid. During supination in CCC, the axis of AST externally rotates and moves laterally relative to the first metatarsal head and sesamoid.

When we find ourselves in static, the 3rd law of Newton, "When a body exerts a force over another, the second always exerts on the first a force of the same magnitude." That is, the force that we provoke in the ground is the same as we receive, this will have a great importance in balancing ground loads and reactive forces. The position that we will have in static is the result of a balance of supination forces medial to the axis and pronating forces lateral to the axis. This example is described by Dr. Kevin Kirby with a seesaw where if the fulcrum is in the middle and the weights of both sides are the same distance and with the same weight should be a balance, just like in a foot where we have an axis of the AST is in neutral.

Subtalar Joint causing Rotational Equilibrium

On the contrary, in a foot where we find a deviated AST axis medially, we will have a seesaw unbalanced where the fulcrum is not found in the center (producing a larger lever arm). This is a simple way to understand that there will be no balance, and another way would be with a higher weight on one edge (like seen in limb length discrepancies). This example helps us understand that a larger lever arm will generate a greater moment. This happens in a foot with a medially deviated AST where we will find that the area of the forefoot will generate a greater moment of pronation than a foot with a normal AST axis.

Practical Biomechanics Question #452: Using the Rotational Equilibrium concept, what is the effect of shortening a lever arm to the rotational force (moment) created?

Practical Biomechanics Question #453: When we think about patients with very pronated medially deviated feet, are the ground reactive forces barefoot generating more supinatory or pronatory moments?

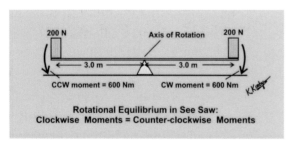

Photo Courtesy of Dr Kevin Kirby showing equal rotational forces on both sides of the

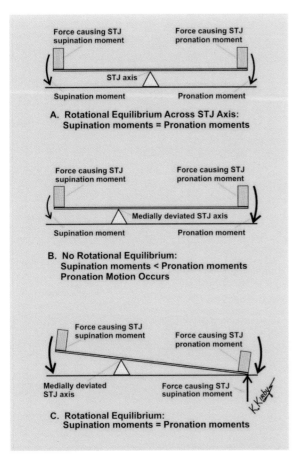

Photo Courtesy of Dr Kevin Kirby with the lower seesaw being corrected by a custom orthotic device to equal the moments

Looking for a seesaw simile, we can compare that edge that when in contact with the ground having the longest lever arm is the limit of pronation in that moment, in the foot that structure would be one or several structures (fascia, tibial posterior, sinus tarsi) that stops pronation depending on the type of foot. This idea is very useful for finding an effective treatment for our patient where we can balance that seesaw. An example would be a Medial Heel Skive in a patient with a syndrome tibialis posterior dysfunction with a AST axis deviated medially where we want to generate a force medial to the axis where we can produce a

supinator moment. Remembering the simile of the seesaw, the more force exerted on the ground that edge of the rocker arm (AST shaft imbalance medially), the more aggressive we should seek treatment to find a balance.

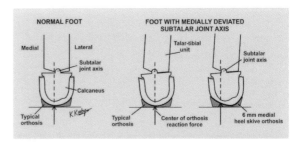

Image Courtesy of Dr Kevin Kirby showing Medial Heel Skive generate a more internal supination moment in a medially deviated subtalar joint axis

Practical Biomechanics Question #454: The medially deviated subtalar joint axis provides a biomechanical challenge in applying appropriate force to help with the over pronation. What are 3 common techniques that accomplish that, and which one seems the most focused on the medial heel area? Answer: 703

On the other side of the balance, on one foot where we find a deviated AST axis laterally, we will have a seesaw unbalanced with the fulcrum also not found in the center (producing a larger lever arm). This imbalance will generate more momentum on one side than the other of the rocker. An example of this lateral deviated axis would be in a patient suffering from peroneal tendonitis, where we find that axis of the AST lateralized. On the rocker would be residing the weight where we have the fulcrum farthest from the center (the edge contacting the ground), where the ground would be the brake of that rotational movement, in this case it would be the peroneal musculature who stopped the movement. Focusing on the treatment as we did in the posterior tibialis dysfunction syndrome earlier, we should add weight in the opposite side to compensate for that balance on the seesaw, or by placing a Lateral Heel Skive to produce a pronating moment.

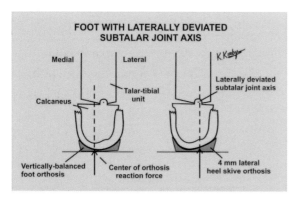

Image Courtesy of Dr Kevin Kirby showing the use of the Lateral Heel Skive in a laterally deviated subtalar joint axis

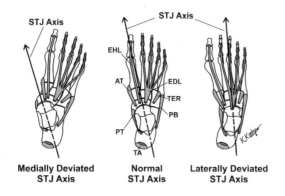

Illustration courtesy of Dr Kevin Kirby showing 3 common placements of the subtalar joint axis. Any ground or orthotic pressure medial to this joint is supinatory and any ground or orthotic pressure lateral to this axis is pronatory.

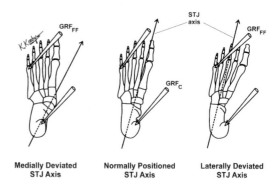

Illustration courtesy of Dr Kevin Kirby showing the typically ground reactive force on the subtalar joint with varying axes

Center of Pressure (COP)

The center of pressure is used often in the study of the function of the foot. Through Dr. Eric A. Fuller in his article "Center of Pressure and Its Theoretical Relationship to Foot Pathology", described a mechanical model that could explain the pathology observed in the foot. He established a relationship between spatial location of the COP and the moments generated on the foot joints; mainly over the subtalar joint.

In order to explain the center of pressure, it is necessary to know what ground reactive forces are. When we walk, gravity exerts a pulling force downward, and this force is countered by another force provided by the ground. This force will have the same magnitude, and opposite direction to that applied by the gravity. This principle is based on newton's third law of action and reaction. These reactive forces act in all areas of the sole of the foot that are in contact with the ground.

These forces located in different areas of the sole of the foot can be grouped at a single point to create a single force, which is equal to the sum of the magnitudes of all the smaller forces. This single point receives the name of the center of pressure, and typically measured by a force plate system.

Practical Biomechanics Question #455: Center of Pressure is a force plate analysis. If you had access to that information, how could CoP and Subtalar Axis position help in your orthotic designs? Answer: 703

It is also the point at which the sum of all these forces generates a zero moment. It is often confused that the center of pressure is the point of maximum pressure. This situation can coincide sometimes. For example, we can get a COP under the head of the second metatarsal, and in turn it can also be the point of maximum pressure. On the contrary, we can find a COP located in the internal longitudinal arch and not having any area of contact with the ground, therefore, having no pressure.

When we walk the COP tends to move through the foot, in the phase of contact is located in the heel, in the middle support phase would be located in the midfoot, and in the toe-off phase in the forefoot.

To describe a force and its relationship with the foot, there are three necessary parameters: location, magnitude and the distance (lever arm) to the axis of movement. The sum of all ground reactive forces generates a vector acting on the foot. Each vector has the ability to generate moments on the joints. In the case of the subtalar joint, if the vector is medial to the axis, it will generate a supinator moment, and if it is lateral to the axis will generate a pronating moment. The moment is the result of the application of a rotational force to an axis. It is determined by the force applied, and by the distance of the location of said force to the axis of movement.

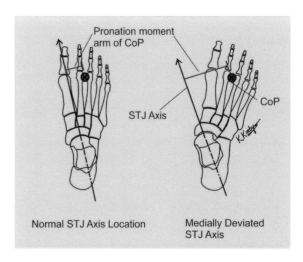

Illustration is courtesy of Dr Kevin Kirby to explain CoP and Pronation Moment Arms

Practical Biomechanics Question #456: There are various forces at play on the foot and rotatory forces having the ability to rotate structures around an axis are called what? And, how is it measured? A: 703

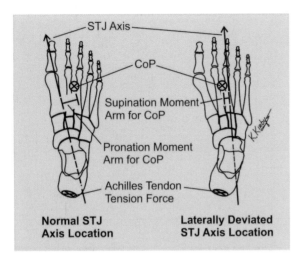

Illustration is courtesy of Dr Kevin Kirby to explain CoP and supination moment arms

Practical Biomechanics Question #457: From the illustration above, the achilles tendon is a natural supinator around the subtalar joint axis attaching medially to that axis. When in gait, does the achilles produce its most powerful subtalar joint supination? Answer: 703

The plantar location of the COP together with the spatial location of the AST axis is used to determine the effects of the mechanics of GRF in AST. You can encounter 3 situations: 1) The COP is located medial to the axis of the AST, 2) The COP is located directly below the axis of the AST, or 3) The COP is located lateral to the axis of the AST. In the event that we find a medialized COP to the axis of the AST, the GRF(s) will cause a supination moment in AST. When the COP is directly below the axis of the AST, there will be no moment produced in the AST since there's no time for the GRF to create a moment throughout the AST axis. When the COP is lateral to the axis of the AST, the GRF will cause a moment of pronation.

It is important to understand distance and COP on which force is exerted with about the AST axis. A major distance will cause greater moment, therefore, greater adaptation of the tissues to find a balance. In the body we have tendons, ligaments, capsules and even joints that resist moments to keep your balance rotational. This concept is very important in the tissue stress approach to biomechanics. In the case of a foot with the axis of the AST deviated more medially, the foot has more chances of developing pathologies in pronation moment resisting structures. In contrast, a foot with AST axis deviated laterally is more likely to have a higher supination moment of GRF and more prone to disease in supination moment resisting structures.

The position of the COP in dynamics is ephemeral, along the path in travels it will go modifying its position both on the axis longitudinal as well as in the transverse axis. And it is that as we walk our AST axis will adapt to the GRF that we generate in the plantar surface of the foot. When the foot pronates in the AST, the axis of the AST internally rotates and moves medially relative to the sole of the foot, so structures of the sole of the foot medial to the axis will cause compression, tissues who perform a supination function will have to be activated, and tissues that control the pronation will have to limit that movement. As the foot supinates in the AST, the axis of the AST rotates externally and moves laterally relative to the sole of the foot, so plantar structures of the foot lateral to the axis will cause a compression, tissues that perform a pronation function will have to be activated, and tissues that control supination will have to limit that movement.

You have to understand the COP and subtalar balance as a marriage, it is not possible that they can coexist without each other. Thanks to COP we can understand why there are patients with a neutral AST axis that suffer from pronator pathology or supinator pathology. The COP solves that unknown, since even having an neutral axis, there may be moments of both supination and pronation in static, or in dynamics, that cause injury to the tissues. In the opposite case, we also find feet in consultation with highly medialized or lateralized axes that remain asymptomatic, situations where the COP lies below that axis, not as medialized or as lateralized, therefore without causing stress in the tissues, since it is in balance.

Practical Biomechanics Question #458: The above implies that a medial deviated subtalar joint axis may not be a powerful pronatory force on the foot due to CoP. Please explain. Answer: 703

Another factor that we have not yet talked about is speed. Sports that are the most explosive tend to be the most harmful. In fact, if a sport has both speed and collusion, they produce the most serious of injuries. Going back to the types of stress that exist, higher compressive stress may be at heel strike up the leg, but this will not have the same stress as the shock of the calcaneus with fat and fascia absorbing that stress. This happens both with walking and running, increasing newtons will cause

more compressive stress with increased speed. This also happens with tensile stress, a patient landing on the forefoot will generate tension in the Achilles when walking, but when running will cause greater tensile stress by increasing the Newtons/m by the increased speed.

Planar Dominance

Pronation is triplanar. It's ordinary to find a deformity in all 3 planes, but normally this deformity is more pronounced in one of the planes, especially in its compensations. This trend has led to the concept of planar dominance, first discussed by Dr Merton Root and colleagues, and then further written about by Dr. Donald Green. Recognizing the plane of the greater deformity component, whether it is sagittal, transverse, or frontal, will allow treatment options to be selected more precisely. The frontal plane deformity can be recognized by a marking increased movement in eversion at the level of the subtalar joint for example. In the transverse plane, pronation recognized by the instability of the talus-navicular joint with medial prominence without excessive heel eversion and no failure of the medial column in the sagittal plane. In the sagittal plane, pronation can be identified because it inverts the posture of the first metatarsal towards dorsiflexion, or the pronation compensation of equinus severely breaks down the medial arch in the sagittal plane (rocker bottom flatfoot). As we understand planar dominance, we can further prevent and reduce devastating compensations.

Practical Biomechanics Question #459: The development of a rocker bottom flatfoot (primarily in the sagittal plane) from an equinus tight achilles condition (primarily a sagittal plane deformity is a great example of this concept of planar dominance. What is a similar planar dominant problem at the knee also caused by equinus forces? 704

Some of the Important Articles for this Chapter

1. Normal and Abnormal Function of the Foot - Clinical Biomechanics Volume II, Root, Merton L.; Weed, John H.; Orien, William P. Published by Clinical Biomechanics Corporation

2. Hicks JH. The mechanics of the foot II. The plantar aponeurosis and the arch. *J Anat.* 1954;88:24-31.

2. Dananberg HJ: Functional hallux limitus and its relationship to gait efficiency. JAPMA 76: 648, 1986.

3. Dananberg HJ: Gait style as an etiology to chronic postural pain: part I. Functional hallux limitus. JAPMA 83:433, 1993.

4. Van Gheluwe B, Dananberg HJ, Hagman F, et al. Effects of hallux limitus on plantar foot pressure and foot kinematics during walking. J Am Podiatr Med Assoc 2006; 96(5): 428–436.

5. Becerro de Bengoa R, Sánchez R, Losa M. Clinical improvement in functional hallux limitus using a cut-out orthosis. Prosthet Orthot Int. 2016 ;40(2): 215-223.

6. Dananberg HJ: Chronic low-back pain and its response to custom-made orthoses. JAPMA 89: 109, 1999.

7. Elftman H, Manter JT. THE AXIS OF THE HUMAN FOOT. *Science.* 1934 Nov 23;80(2082):484–484

8. Van Langelaan EJ. A kinematical analysis of the tarsal joints. An X-ray photogrammetric study. Acta Orthop Scand Suppl. 1983;204:1-269.
9. Christopher J Nester , Andrew H Findlow, Clinical and experimental models of the midtarsal joint: proposed terms of reference and associated terminology. J Am Podiatr Med Assoc. 2006 Jan-Feb;96(1):24-31.

10. McPoil TG, Hunt GC. Evaluation and management of foot and ankle disorders: Present problems and future directions. *J Orthop Sports Phys Ther.* 1995; 21(6):381-388.

11. Kirby, KA, Subtalar joint axis location and rotational equilibrium theory of foot function, J Am Podiatr Med Assoc, 2001 Oct;91(9):465-87

12. Kirby, KA: The medial heel skive technique. Improving pronation control in foot orthoses. J Am Podiatr Med Assoc. 1992 Apr;82(4):177-88.
13. Fuller, E.A. Center of pressure and its theoretical relationship to foot pathology. JAPMA, 89:278-91, 1999.

14. Green DR, Carol A. Planal dominance.
J Am Podiatry Assoc.1984
Feb;74(2):98–103.

Chapter 9: Pronation and Supination Syndromes

FOOT SUPINATION AND PRONATION

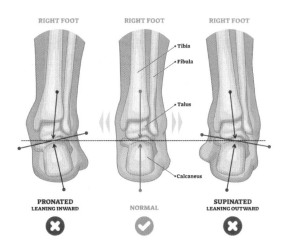

I spend my whole life trying to make patients more stable. I get a few athletes still that only want just that---to be more stable in hopes it will help their performance. I am afraid that the barefoot movement has ruined that part of my practice with its teaching of shoe and orthotic freedom. Fortunately, most of my patients really only want to feel better. They are plagued by injuries, or just pain areas, and they seek my advice, and the advice of thousands of dedicated podiatrists, physical therapists, chiropractors, medical doctors, trainers, etc. In fact, there are over 40 or 50 professional organizations that have a sports medicine branch. These organizations are all trying to help athletes, and non-athletes alike, feel better. Each profession has a range of treatment options for these patients that come into their offices, and I hope this book which touches on mechanical treatments

adequately describes what Podiatry has to offer. Remember my mantra is "Stability begets Comfort".

This chapter summarizes how the abnormal motions of excessive pronation and contact phase supination can cause problems at the foot and up the chain. I am always asking my patients how the orthotic devices are working and what symptoms are improved, and what symptoms are not (or even made worse) by the most recent changes I made. The foot orthotic world wants to go back to the 1950s and 60s when the belief was that there was only one perfect orthotic device for any one individual. That has been proven incorrect in my office daily where any single biomechanical problem (like forefoot varus), placed into 5 different pairs of shoes, or participated in 5 different activities, could require different supports for each to make the athlete comfortable and stable. Shoes and activities vary so much that they eternally need to be customized. However, the patient will still have some structural faults like bow legs that will not change, and functional faults like weak and tight muscles and upslipped sacro-iliac joints that maybe can change, and it makes helping these patients in their real life so both challenging and rewarding, frustrating at times, and incredibly fulfilling at other times.

The fact that there is so much variability offered in biomechanical treatments should be looked at as sent from the heavens, but I am afraid it produces a daunting task for some/most. So, I am here to teach you solid rules in this book that can bring the fun back to this part of the practice of medicine, if it wasn't already there. Learn the principles of a mechanical approach to injuries and pain syndromes, and it will also help your surgical practice, and your wound care practice, etc. This book is a reflection of my life's work and I hope it can inspire future generations.

Practical Biomechanics Question #460: As we begin to discuss Over Pronation Syndrome, what are the various types of over pronation treated (a wide range of answers are accepted)? Answer: 704

Over Pronation Syndrome

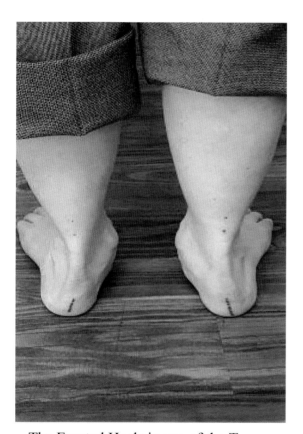

The Everted Heels is one of the Top Measurements Made to Document the Amount of Pronation

I will start with abnormal pronation. What is abnormal pronation when pronation is good for shock absorption and our adaptability to the ground? If pronation is good during the contact phase of gait, why is it bad?

The problem lies in the duration of the pronation (into midstance and propulsion), the speed of the pronation (making it harder for muscles to decelerate that motion), and the position the pronation leaves the patient. I like the concept that the patient is not properly stacked up as in the photo image just preceding. The injuries listed below could be from many factors, and be part of what I call the Biomechanics Rule of 3 (as discussed in Chapters 1 and 2 of Book 1). This rule states that it can take 3 biomechanical problems to cause a problem in the first place leaving the area to be injured vulnerable. It creates a weak link in the patient's chain of armor. Any one of the 3 factors (and it could be more like 5-6) can be the most important to correct improving the speed of recovery and the prevention of recurrence of the same injury. I suggest that pronation can be the main cause of the below problems, or just an aggravating factor in healing, and therefore learning how to correct pronation is important.

Practical Biomechanics Question #461: Using the Rule of 3, what are common biomechanical causes of tibial sesamoid stress that should be evaluated and treated if found? Answer: 704

Practical Biomechanics Question #462: Using the Rule of 3, what are common biomechanical causes of 4th metatarsal stress that should be evaluated and treated if found? Answer: 704

Practical Biomechanics Question #463: Using the Rule of 3, what are common biomechanical causes of peroneal tendon stress on the lateral ankle area that should be evaluated and treated if found? A: 704

The motion of pronation itself is partly for shock absorption. We need to pronate when we strike the ground to absorb shock. The motion the foot makes as it pronates is a very efficient shock absorber. Pronation at heel contact is part of normal motion. The motion of pronation also loosens the foot to adapt to the ground. If you have ever held a foot at the heel and moved the forefoot, you can see the fascinating difference of motion when the heel is inverted maximally (supinated) versus everted maximally (pronated). The entire foot moves so much more when you are pronated at the subtalar joint than when you are supinated at the subtalar joint. This is why forefoot deformities are measured with the subtalar joint in a neutral position. There always has to be a reference point. Movement away from this subtalar neutral position will greatly influence the position of the forefoot to rearfoot. The motion of pronation is also important to continue the internal rotation of the leg. In the swing phase, the leg changes directions from externally rotating in mid stance and propulsion to internally rotating with swing and contact phases of gait. These are the normal transverse plane motions of the lower extremity, and contact phase internal rotation with foot pronation are both normal and important to the motion of the whole leg. These are important functions of pronation when it occurs at the contact phase of gait. When pronation does not occur, or occurs too much, problems can develop.

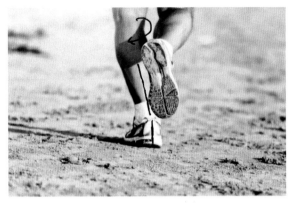

This image illustrates when the leg internal rotation, with heel eversion, is happening too long (well into the beginning of propulsion of the weight bearing foot)

The problems with pronation that podiatrists work on daily is when it is too much, not enough, or happening at the wrong time. The too much part means that it is more than the normal amount of pronation, or happening too quickly. The not enough can occur when a foot is already maximally pronated, and so does not have the pronation motion at heel contact. The happening at the wrong time part means that the pronation continues through the contact phase into midstance, or has contact phase supination with late midstance pronation, or just has propulsive phase pronation. Let's look some at each of these situations

Practical Biomechanics Question #464: What is a common example of pronation only occurring in late midstance? A: 704

Typically when pronation is too much at heel contact it keeps the leg internally rotated up to the propulsive phase. It is only with lifting the heel off of the ground that propulsive phase supination can occur letting the lower leg externally rotate to catch up to the upper thigh area. This integral relationship is observed with the help of knee rotation. We watch the knee internally rotate during the contact phase, stay internally rotated in the mid stance, and then in propulsion start to externally rotate some.

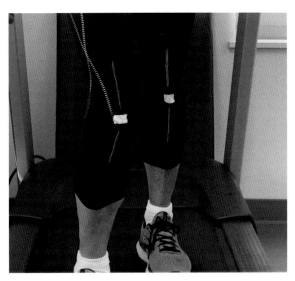

This image showing the knee staying internally rotated well past the contact phase

Typically when pronation happens too quickly, this ballistic motion can be very damaging to the body. I see it on a few patients walking, and more commonly tied to the running motion.

Practical Biomechanics Question #465: Many times this sport specific pronation is not seen in walking gait evaluation or indicated in their biomechanical examinations. What modification is essential in a custom insert for this problem? Answer: 704

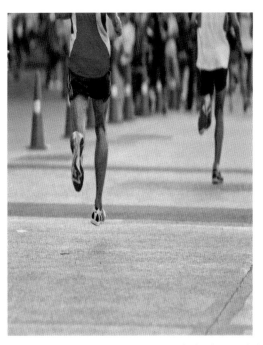

This image demonstrates a right lateral foot strike very inverted which will rapidly pronate the foot and produce pronatory moments up the leg

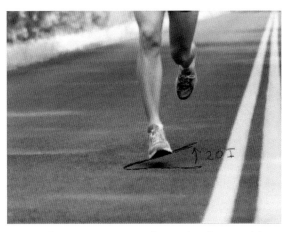

Another runner seen from the front with estimated 20 degrees of inverted foot strike causing rapid foot pronation

It can be related to a sharp edge to the subtalar joint axis that falls into pronation quickly. It can be related to weak medial muscles that should be decelerating this motion following heel contact. It can simply be related to some shoe design or orthotic/shoe interface that causes the patient to hit the lateral corner in a heel inverted, and then to be catapulted into pronation. If an orthotic device is involved, by having the patient walk and/or run with and without their orthotic devices they will look worse with my devices. As an experiment, I can easily remove the rearfoot post to see if it smoothes the transition medially following heel contact. I may also have them make an appointment and bring in 3-4 pairs of shoes to see which one gives the smoothest flow of motion.

Practical Biomechanics Question #466: What would you expect to see if a patient brought in 3 pairs of shoes (neutral, stability, and maximal control) and you could watch the same orthotic device in each? Answer: 704

Practical Biomechanics Question #467: What would you expect to see if a patient brought in 3 pairs of shoes (all neutral but zero drop, moderate heel drop, and maximal heel drop) and you could watch the same orthotic device in each? Answer: 704

Typically when pronation is not enough, the foot is already pronated maximally, or the foot is being held in supination. You can also get the patients that your subtalar joint range of motion examination showed marked limitation of overall motion

(perhaps tarsal coalition). For the patients that are functioning in maximal pronation, you can see this commonly in these types of problems:

1. Rearfoot valgus or rigid flat feet (from equinus, congenital conditions, some PTTD conditions, genu valgum, etc.)
2. High rear foot varus deformities (like genu or tibial varum) which stay maximally pronated, instead of resupinating, likely due to the energy required to resupinate with every step.
3. Limited subtalar joint range of motion (possible tarsal coalition).

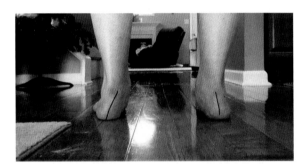

Everted heels functioning maximally pronated (as shown in the Maximum Pronation Test in Chapter 4)

Typically when pronation happens at the wrong time, it is related to these conditions that typically leave the medial column unstable:

1. The pronation of heel strike continues into the midstance and possibly the propulsive phase of gait.
2. With many cases of contact phase lateral instability, like with flexible or rigid forefoot valgus, the subtalar joint needs to pronate in late

midstance to move the body medially for propulsion.

3. In some cases of rearfoot varus and forefoot varus, the subtalar joint can only pronate enough for the rearfoot varus leaving the medial forefoot off of the ground until propulsion where there is a collapse medially as weight attempts to go to the first metatarsal. This is seen with metatarsus primus elevatus also.

Here is a list of foot and lower extremity problems that I give to my students that can be caused by excessive pronation. The list was generated by various articles, but mainly years of evaluation of what symptoms could improve if I corrected for excessive pronation. The list for pronation is founded on the concepts produced by over pronation: medial instability, excessive rotation or torque on various structures, poor shock absorption if you are fully pronated, increased medial foot weight bearing, if the pronation blocks the normal forward motion of the foot in gait, and lateral knee weight bearing. There is a summary of problems related to excessive pronation. They include:

1. First Metatarsal Phalangeal Joint Pain
2. Sesamoid Injuries
3. Bunions
4. Second Metatarsal Phalangeal Joint Capsulitis
5. Metatarsalgia
6. Second Metatarsal Stress Fractures
7. Morton's Neuroma or Neuritis
8. Hammertoes
9. Intrinsic Muscle Strain
10. Plantar Fasciitis
11. Anterior Tibial Tendonitis
12. Lateral sinus tarsitis
13. Cuboid Syndrome
14. Lateral Ankle Impingement
15. Posterior Tibial Injuries
16. Tarsal Tunnel Syndrome
17. Peroneus Longus Strain
18. Achilles Strain
19. Tibial Stress Fractures
20. Medial Soleus Strain
21. Lateral Knee Compartment Syndrome
22. Pes Anserinus Tendonitis/Bursitis
23. Patellofemoral Injuries
24. Anterior Cruciate Injuries
25. Medial Hamstring Strains
26. Iliotibial Band Syndrome
27. Piriformis Syndrome
28. Low Back Pain

Practical Biomechanics Question #468: People have weak spots. Dr Blake uses a Rule of 3 to discover 2 other (and perhaps more) problems leading to an injury if over pronation is listed as one of the causes. What would be 2 other common causes of second metatarsal stress fracture? A: 705

First metatarsal phalangeal joint pain can develop with or without functional hallux limitus. The big toe joint is the end of the medial column, and part of the essential tripod of foot support. Increase in stress and pain is commonly seen in a long first metatarsal, but not necessarily. Big toe joint pain can be caused by overpronation which overloads the big toe joint as the weight shifts excessively medially. This can eliminate the joint's ability to push off, even for milliseconds, which can irritate the low back. Over pronation causes overall looseness in the tissues increasing the chance that the joint functions improperly. Treatment of big toe joint pain should start by treating the over pronation of the foot dramatically reducing the stresses on the big toe joint.

Sesamoid Injuries can be caused by overpronation injuring the sesamoids with the medial shift in body weight. This is commonly seen with pes cavus foot type, plantar flexed first rays, and bi-partite sesamoids, which are three other biomechanical factors. The goal of custom foot orthotic devices would be to shift weight back into the arch, and also shift the weight laterally into the 2nd and 3rd metatarsals more during the propulsive phase.

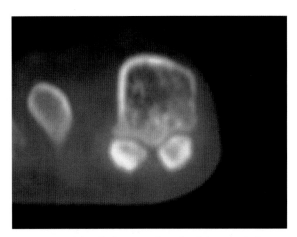

Sesamoids sitting under the big toe joint

Bunions are produced as the chronic nature of pronation overloading the medial side of the foot causes instability of the first metatarsal first cuneiform joint. This then leads to slow first metatarsal drift in

abduction, inversion, and dorsiflexion directions. This is also commonly seen with metatarsus adductus, ligamentous laxity, rounded first metatarsal heads, short first metatarsals, metatarsus primus elevatus, etc. Patients with over pronation can have normal big toe joint alignment, so many factors are involved. Tight shoes usually are involved with the advancement from Stage 2 to Stage 3 or 3 to 4, but not in the early signs of formation.

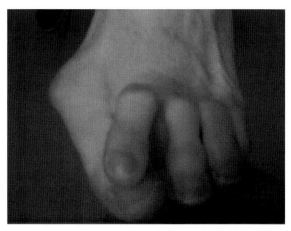

Stage 4 Bunion totally destabilizes the medial column and makes it very different to walk well

Practical Biomechanics Question #469: Remember to always make a patient more stable. What is the Stage of Bunion development that surgery should be at least considered? Answer: 705

Second metatarsal phalangeal joint capsulitis can be caused by overpronation which moves the weight of the body medially, putting too much pressure on the second metatarsal. Of course, this will occur if the first metatarsal is not able to take enough weight when the second metatarsal is too long, or congenitally too low, or recently dropped, or metatarsus primus elevatus exists. This will either slowly or acutely cause a plantar plate issue and hammertoe development. If there is a bunion, and the 2nd joint needs an operation, the bunion is corrected also.

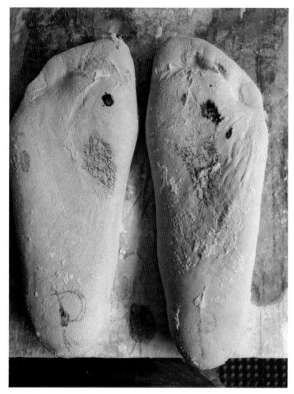

These are typical impression casts. The low spots are marked with black, so you can see that the left foot has a metatarsus primus elevatus with more weight under the 2nd metatarsal

Practical Biomechanics Question #470: Chronic overload of the 2nd MPJ due to over pronation can lead to what injuries?

Metatarsalgia can be caused by overpronation which is a tri-planar motion causing excessive shear and torque as the forefoot experiences the ground reactive forces pushing up on the metatarsal heads of

inversion, dorsiflexion, and abduction. Over pronation loosens the foot more than it should be in the later part of stance. These abnormal forces are typically related to late midstance or propulsive pronation, and accompanied with forefoot abduction on the rearfoot (but that depends on the orientation of the joint axes). Instead of the forefoot firmly accepting the body's weight at heel lift, the forefoot slides around increasing shear forces and overall abnormal forces. All cases of metatarsalgia typically treated must have any achilles tightness resolved and metatarsal collapse supported with a variety of metatarsal pads, even when custom orthotic devices are made.

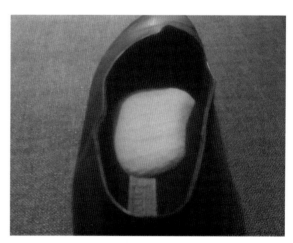

This is a typical large metatarsal support used in metatarsal problems from Hapad ®

Second metatarsal stress fractures can be caused by overpronation which will move weight bearing medially. There are situations where the second metatarsal may be stressed due to its position alone, or that the first metatarsal does not accept enough load. Again, this is typically seen with bunions and long second metatarsals and toes (Morton's Foot). I am always trying to find out why pronation did not transfer weight all the way across to the first metatarsal avoiding the second metatarsal.

Practical Biomechanics Question #471: Summarize in which situations why the motion of over pronation ends up hurting the 2nd metatarsal and not the first or just medial column. Answer: 705

Morton's Neuroma

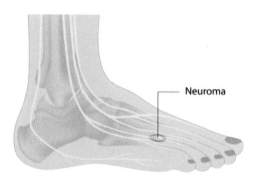

Neuroma

Morton's neuromas or neuritis can be caused by overpronation in late midstance or propulsion. This abnormal motion will cause some cuboid and fourth and fifth metatarsal instability. The classic Morton's Neuroma is caused by irritation of the nerve at the junction of the medial and lateral plantar nerves. The overpronation causes excessive motion of the 4th metatarsal (linked to the cuboid) on the more stable 3rd metatarsal, although even the 3rd metatarsal is moving. Any other problem with the sciatic nerve, like heel eversion pulling on the posterior tibial nerve at the medial ankle, or internal femoral rotation tightening the fibres of the piriformis muscle on the sciatic nerve, or the low back straightening due to tight hamstrings developing from over pronation and

increased knee flexion, can cause increased neural tension and pain at various trigger points.

Practical Biomechanics Question #472: How does a tight achilles tendon, which can cause abnormal pronation, also produce excessive pressure on the metatarsals leading to nerve hypersensitivity? A: 705

Hammertoes can have their root in any instability of the foot. Overpronation in the contact phase is important to loosen up the foot and allow it to adapt to a variety of surfaces. However, when the pronated loose packed foot stays pronated during the midstance and propulsion, stability is lost in the midfoot, so the toes claw the ground for stability. Other causes of instability, whether related to pronation or not, which can increase the hammering of toes: pes cavus with medial or lateral instability, weak achilles tendons with over firing of the FHL and FDL tendons to help lift the heel, weak quadriceps, poor eyesight and the need to grip more, etc.

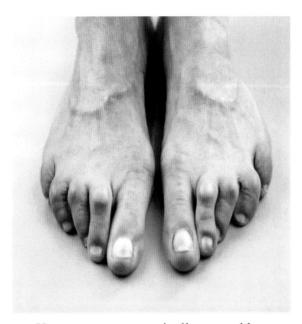

Hammertoes are typically caused by instabilities, one by an over pronated loose foot trying to gain stability

Intrinsic muscle strain can be caused by overpronation as the foot flattens the arch and stresses the intrinsic muscles. The intrinsic muscles have to work overtime stabilizing the foot, especially the digits at propulsion. They can easily strain in an overuse situation, like walking more than normal in non supportive shoes. This can also happen when wearing shoes that the toes have to grip to keep you from coming out of the shoes. The more pronated the foot, and the looser and more unstable the ligaments, the intrinsic muscles have to work harder to keep the patient upright. The best exercises for the intrinsics are metatarsal doming since they do not encourage digital flexion leading to hammertoes.

Plantar fasciitis can be caused by overpronation. This problem is probably the most talked about of all pronatory problems as it is one of the most common injuries of the foot. The foot pronates too much, and the arch collapses too much. This puts a stretch on the plantar fascia causing a first degree sprain of this important ligament, especially with medial overload of the first metatarsal head. This is especially true since the plantar fascia does not stretch much at all, regarded as not too adaptable. The plantar fascia, a ligament, is designed to undergo high tensile and shear stresses, but can be still overloaded. High arched feet, with a tighter plantar fascia, when they pronate too much can develop very recalcitrant cases of plantar fasciitis. If you were just to look at the non-weight bearing structure of feet that get plantar fasciitis, most would have normal to high arched feet. Middle age patients can develop plantar fascial tears (second or third degree sprains) due to a lifetime of insult to the plantar fascial fibers and resultant degenerative changes called plantar fasciosis. This same insult can lead to a slow development of calcaneal spurs.

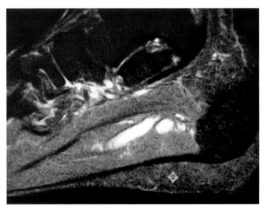

MRI of a solid plantar fascia with the sensor below originating at the heel bone

Practical Biomechanics Question #473: The plantar fascia is a tertiary support for our feet. Over pronation of the foot can cause instability of the primary ligaments, thus making the intrinsic muscles work harder. Theorize how this scenario could place stress on the plantar fascia especially if the intrinsic muscles were not strong. (705)

Anterior tibial tendonitis can be caused by overpronation. The anterior tibial tendon decelerates both the foot at heel contact to slow down foot slap (its dorsiflexion or extension function), and it decelerates overall rearfoot pronation (its frontal plane function). When the velocity of rearfoot pronation is high, as in runners or other athletes, or the foot is very pronated at push-off in walkers, the anterior tibial tendon gets overused. It can also be one of the first signs the foot is developing adult acquired flatfoot, so watch these patients carefully. Anterior tibial symptoms can also develop when the posterior ankle structures are tight making it harder to work to dorsiflex the foot.

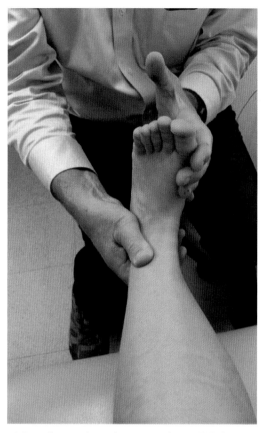

Muscle testing the Anterior Tibial Tendon by having the patient Dorsiflex and then Invert and then applying gradual pressure to evert

Lateral sinus tarsitis, also called sinus tarsi syndrome, can be caused by over pronation. This over pronation typically has to involve marked heel eversion and seen a lot in athletes due to their high volume of pronation. With closed kinetic chain subtalar joint pronation, the calcaneus everts on the inverting, or relatively stationary, talus. This sets up the lateral subtalar joint for impingement problems, while over stretching the medial side of the joint.

Cuboid syndrome can be caused by an acute inversion sprain discussed under oversupination, but can also be caused by overpronation. The stabilization of the cuboid is one of the most important functions of the achilles tendon (gastrocnemius and soleus) in the contact phase. Upon heel contact, with the heel inverted, the firing of the gastrocnemius and soleus traps the cuboid against the ground in a stable position. The cuboid must be stable against the ground to allow for the re-supination of the subtalar joint at mid stance partially through the firing of the peroneus longus that anchors under the cuboid. With over pronation, the cuboid remains unstable, and it can get jammed in abnormal positions helped with mobilization techniques and orthotic devices to reduce the overall pronation.

Practical Biomechanics Question #474: An unstable cuboid renders the peroneal tendon utterly useless. Explain why stabilizing the cuboid, even if it requires an Inverted Orthotic Device, can make the lateral ankle so much more stable. Answer: 705

Lateral ankle impingement is similar to lateral sinus tarsitis and can be caused by overpronation. This is most commonly seen in sports where the rapid heel eversion with subtalar joint pronation can produce impingement pain between lateral border of talus and medial border of the tip of the fibula (even causing stress fractures of the fibula). Since it is lateral, it is often misdiagnosed as peroneal tendonitis or lateral ankle instability, and treatments like ankle braces to force the foot into pronation are used unsuccessfully.

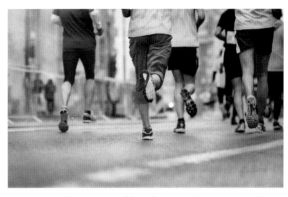

Various degrees of heel eversion excursion is noted in this one photo from mild to severe (which is what is needed for lateral ankle impingement)

Posterior tibial injuries including accessory navicular syndrome is a common sports injury caused by over pronation, and an ominous sign that an adult acquired flat foot may be coming in non-athletes. The posterior tibial tendon is the most important, and most direct, decelerator of subtalar joint pronation, and support on the medial longitudinal arch. I would say it is the most important protector of the spring ligament. The anatomy of the posterior tibial tendon complex makes it one of the best examples of how the body will hurt at the weakest link in the chain. It is easy to understand how overpronation can produce stress on the posterior tibial tendon which will fight hard to reduce the overall pronation or speed of pronation. But where will it hurt? The posterior tibial when stressed will hurt at its weakest link. If the tibia, at its origin is weak, a tibial stress fracture can occur. If the weakest link is the periosteum, then shin splints occur. If the muscle belly is the weak link, then myositis or calf strain is diagnosed. If the tendon is the weak link, then tendonitis occurs (stage I to III). If there is an accessory navicular, that may be the weak spot, and os navicularis syndrome occurs. If the fibres of the tendon that go into the arch are the weak spots, then arch pain occurs. One motion, one anatomical structure, 6-7 places of potential pain.

Practical Biomechanics Question #475: If there is an accessory navicular, when did it fully form and how much of the posterior tibial tendon attaches into it instead of the navicular bone? Answer: 705

Tarsal tunnel syndrome can be caused by overpronation. Overpronation of the foot at the ankle can cause a stretching of the medial ankle structures for a prolonged or exaggerated timeframe when the heel is everted. This can even occur with a vertical heel position when there is a high degree of tibial varum and the subtalar joint is pronated many degrees from its neutral position. This over stretching or pulling on the medial structures can cause an entrapment or chronic irritation of the posterior tibial nerve under the laciniate ligament. Secondarily, if this same pronation causes one of the 3 tendons in the tarsal tunnel to develop some form of tendon strain with swelling the posterior tibial nerve can become irritated by that chronic swelling. All 3 tendons, posterior tibial, flexor hallucis longus, and flexor digitorum longus are pronatory decelerators at heel contact. There are cases where the muscle belly of one of the 3 tendons extends into the tarsal tunnel causing entrapment due to muscle hypertrophy in

trying to decelerate excessive pronation. If you add any other cause of nerve irritation, whether proximal or distal, the tarsal tunnel symptoms get worse. What then is the best position mechanically for the tarsal tunnel? That position would be where the subtalar joint is as close to neutral so that there are equal stresses on both the medial and lateral tissues. The subtalar neutral can be inverted in tibial varum cases, vertical at times, and everted in genu valgum/tibial valgum cases.

Peroneus longus strain can be caused by overpronation. The peroneus longus has many functions, but one is to attach to the plantar surface of the first metatarsal base and plantar flex the first metatarsal in resupination, especially at push off. When excessive pronation overloads the medial side of the foot, jamming the first metatarsal upwards or dorsiflexed to the first cuneiform (also called hypermobile first ray), making the peroneus longus work very hard, and many times failing to plantar flex the first metatarsal. Proper smooth propulsion of the foot can not occur, and peroneus longus tendon strain occurs. Typically you are in a functional hallux limitus situation. Since the peroneus longus also protects the lateral ankle, we will see it mentioned as caused by oversupination also. The above scenario is made so impossible by the overpronation causing instability at the cuboid. An unstable cuboid means anchoring of the peroneus longus is very difficult adding to its inability to plantar flex the first metatarsal for propulsion.

Practical Biomechanics Question #476: If abnormal excessive pronation causes the foot to become a loose bag of bones (some more than others), which destabilizes the cuboid, how would you summarize its effects on the peroneus longus tendon, the first ray, and the lateral ankle? A: 705

Achilles strain can be caused by overpronation. I first heard discussion on the achilles tendon and pronation in 1979 in a lecture from Dr. Steven Subotnick. The achilles is the most powerful tendon in the body moving up to 11 times body weight in the sagittal plane. Like the quadriceps and hamstrings, it is primarily a sagittal plane mover. Excessive pronation can cause both excessive frontal plane and transverse plane twists or torques on the tendon that can cause tendon strain. In designing an orthotic device for achilles strain patients, I try to see if I can place the resting heel position closer to the neutral heel position. Since orthotic devices affect all three planes, even with primarily frontal plane corrections, the transverse plane twisting can be reduced. I want the achilles to be functioning in the sagittal plane as much as possible.

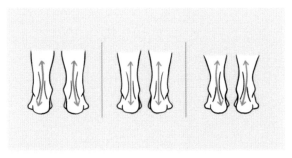

The center illustration is functioning in the sagittal plane, the pronated left and supinated right have to function with more stress thus strain more easily

Tibial stress fractures can be caused by overpronation. This overpronation causes excessive internal tibial rotation. Some of the biggest muscles that decelerate this pronation attach on the tibia, especially the posterior tibial and soleus. The pull can be so great (based on the activity of the patient) that the tibia can break. The tibia can be somewhat weakened with Vitamin D deficiency, or poor bone density, making this bone the weakest link in the chain. The tibia on a standing x-ray can have significant curves where stress points along the bone can occur in the convex or concave parts. Since knee motion can be dependent or independent on foot motion, there are many individuals that have tremendous foot pronation with no patellar internal rotation. In these situations, the torque that naturally goes up the leg into the knee and hip, is stopped in the tibia or knee abruptly leading to tibial stress. Remember the stress point is where there is motion after relative immobility. This can occur with an ankle brace limiting ankle motion but putting the stress above or below.

Practical Biomechanics Question #477: What is the strongest muscle attaching into the tibia that decelerates subtalar joint pronation? Answer: 706

Medial soleus strain, like posterior tibial pain, can be caused by overpronation. The soleus is part of the two muscles that make up the achilles tendon. It originates from both the proximal aspects of the posterior tibia and posterior fibula. It not only works to plantar flex the ankle at push off, but supinates the subtalar joint to help with the overall external leg rotation of the lower extremity. If the foot is held in a prolonged pronated position into the propulsive phase, or if the foot pronates in the late midstance or propulsive phases, the soleus fibers can stress and muscle strain occurs. And, since it is active right after heel contact to trap the cuboid down, it is a good muscle to attempt to decelerate overpronation during the early milliseconds following heel contact.

Practical Biomechanics Question #478: The discussion above was on the stress to decelerate over pronation placed on the soleus. What are 2 common reasons found in our biomechanical examinations which analyze possible soleus weakness which would make it strain easier? Answer: 706

Lateral knee compartment injury can be caused or aggravated by over pronation. It is easy to use the general rule that pronation causes medial foot and medial lower extremity symptoms, and supination causes lateral foot and lateral lower extremity symptoms, but there are so many exceptions like lateral knee compartment injuries. When I first started to work in an orthopedic clinic at Saint Francis Memorial Hospital in San Francisco, Dr. James Garrick, world renowned orthopedist, had me treat all the medial and lateral meniscal injuries that were either not appropriate for surgery at the time, post op to relieve pressure off the operated knee joint compartment, or just when the patient wanted to try as much conservative treatment as was reasonable. In straight forward logic, if you had lateral meniscal

issues, you would want to open up and decompress the lateral compartment by varus wedging the foot. This worked so well on half of the patients that 35 plus years later some of these same patients have still avoided surgery and are asking me to make them more wedges on an annual basis. But, the knee joint is influenced by not only foot motion, but by the knee's own axis of motion, and by hip motion. Therefore, 50% of patients did not respond to lateral wedging, but everyone seemed to be helped by some form of foot stability correction. Of course, this would never happen if their knee locked or kept buckling where surgery was more apparent.

Practical Biomechanics Question #479: Over pronation of the foot compresses which side of the knee joint? Answer: 706

Pes anserinus tendinitis/bursitis is caused by overpronation in runners primarily. The pes anserinus, meaning goose feet, is the conjoined tendons of 3 muscles attaching into the proximal medial aspect of the anterior tibia for stabilization at foot contact of the knee. The three muscles are the sartorius, gracilis, and semitendinosus, also called guy ropes, and the mnemonic SGT can help you remember. By their attachment, at foot strike, and it is primarily a running related injury, it stabilizes the anterior medial knee area which is stressed in the overpronation motion of excessive internal tibial rotation on the femur. It protects the anterior cruciate ligament which is trying to stop the anterior and medial displacement of the tibia on the femur from inside the knee. I especially see it injured during downhill running, where these medial knee structures have to stabilize a flexing knee at foot strike where the force can be 10 times body weight.

Patellofemoral injuries can be caused by overpronation of the foot. This is one of the most common injuries in all sports, and has a myriad of acronyms like quadriceps insufficiency, runner's knee, biker's knee, dancer's knee, chondromalacia patellae, patellofemoral dysfunction, etc. The problem lies in the kneecap or patella not staying in its normal femoral groove, but slides laterally thus irritating the medial aspect of the posterior surface of the patella. This lateral subluxation is helped with taping the patella slightly medially, bracing the patella to hold it more centered (you see braces with the kneecap hole), strengthening the vastus medialis and external hip rotators, and stretching the very powerful vastus lateralis to weaken its pull laterally. With overpronation, sometimes just produced by the sport in a normal foot, 2 mechanisms can be to blame either fully or partially. If the overpronation causes the knee to assume a more valgus position of the tibia on the femur, this alignment causes the vastus lateralis to have more power pulling the patella laterally (also called the Q angle or Quadriceps angle). If the overpronation simply produces more internal rotation of the tibia on the femur, the vastus lateralis is placed in tone, and the vastus medialis relaxed creating a dynamic muscle imbalance leading again to the lateral subluxation of the patella. This, along with many injuries above the foot,

requires a varus angulation placed into the shoe, as a wedge or as an orthotic device. This wedging can later be reduced or eliminated in the future if not needed.

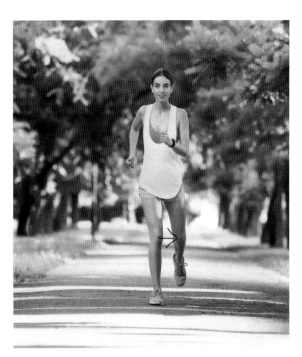

Internal hip rotation with pronation can place the knee too internal with the vastus lateralis pulling the kneecap laterally out of its normal groove

Practical Biomechanics Question #480: Patellofemoral injuries was one of the first sports knee injuries that Podiatrists were treating with great success in the 1970s. Explain how the internal rotation of the limb increases the power of the vastus lateralis. Answer: 706

Anterior Cruciate Injuries can be helped by devices that stop overpronation. Whereas I do not think that ACL injuries are caused by overpronation, but from our previous discussion of pes anserinus injuries, the anterior cruciate ligament functions to stop both anterior motion of the tibia on the femur and internal rotation of the tibia on the femur. When treating patients with ACL injuries, either conservatively or post operatively, custom orthotics or simply varus wedges that can control the internal rotation of the tibia on the femur can take a great deal of stress away from the ACL. I have used this for hundreds of patients to help in their knee rehabilitation.

Practical Biomechanics Question #481: Flat feet has been proposed as a precursor to some ACL tears, since it preloads the ligament as the foot abnormally pronates. If abnormal foot pronation places the knee more internal and flexed, why would that put stress on the ACL ligament? A: 706

Medial hamstring strains that are chronic in nature can be caused by overpronation. The medial hamstrings are the semimembranosus, attaching into the posterior medial aspect of the proximal tibia, and the semitendinosus, part of the pes anserinus, attaching into the anterior medial aspect of the proximal tibia. In normal function, the medial hamstrings are knee flexors and internal rotators of the tibia helping with foot pronation. However, with excessive foot pronation, the role of the semitendinosus as part of the pes anserinus must be to protect the anterior medial knee and stop the forward motion of the tibia. This repeated motion can cause strain of the medial hamstrings especially when the hamstrings are weakened by excessive tightness.

Practical Biomechanics Question #482A: There are 2 medial and 2 lateral hamstrings. Please name them and explain why tight hamstrings strain easier than normal length hamstrings. Answer: 706

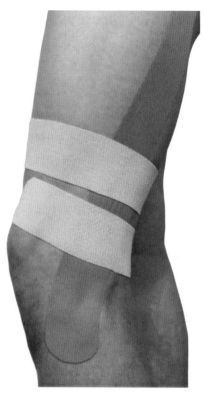

Classic ITB taping, blue to reinforce, green (pulled anterior to posterior in tension) to limit anterior excursion with overpronation across the lateral femoral epicondyle

Iliotibial band syndrome can have overpronation as one of its causes. One of my most favorite structures is the ITB. Its primary function is to protect the lateral hip and the lateral knee at foot strike. Like the plantar fascia, it is mainly fascia tissue, so it is very hard but not impossible to stretch. Conventionally you can get a good stretch proximally at its origin in the tensor fascia lata and gluteus medius fibers. But, rolling with an ethafoam roller of the fascial fibers does help. It is a very common running injury and it does not take alot to cause it to be overworked. Excessive pronation is only one motion that can irritate it, but probably the most publicized. As the femur internally rotates with excessive subtalar joint pronation, the tibia, where the iliotibial band attaches, internally rotates more relative to the femur. This motion of internal rotation tibia on the femur brings the iliotibial band anterior over two body landmarks. These landmarks are the greater trochanters around the hip area and the lateral femoral epicondyles at the knee. Women typically develop ITBS at the hips and men at the knees, but this is a generalization with many exceptions. We will discuss later how oversupination can cause this problem also.

Piriformis syndrome can be caused by overpronation. With walking and running, the piriformis is an external hip rotator. Therefore, excessive pronation which causes excessive internal hip rotation strains the piriformis muscle trying to decelerate that internal motion. The interesting and perplexing aspect of piriformis syndrome is how it can involve the sciatic nerve and cause neurological symptoms. The sciatic nerve can run under, over, or between the fibers of the piriformis. So many problems we treat have a neuropathic aspect because the sciatic nerve gets irritated. You can get classic sciatica symptoms, or just vague neuropathic symptoms, and maybe some hip symptoms.

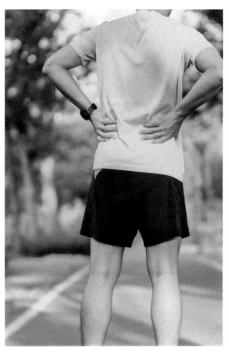

It is very important to discuss with back pain when they get pain: walking, sitting, laying, or only doing certain movements

Low Back symptoms is the last I will discuss under overpronation. The classic cause, as taught to the world by Dr Howard Dananberg, is the restriction of forward motion caused by over pronation. This is caused by the dorsiflexed position of the first metatarsal due to pronatory forces, thus limiting the ability of the first metatarsal to plantar flex in active push off. The momentary restriction of the body to move forward can chronically stress the low back. This chronic stress to the low back can eventually lead to pain.

Practical Biomechanics Question #482B: Name the 28 injuries or pain areas that can be caused or aggravated by over pronation. This implies that treatment of that over pronation may reduce or eliminate present symptoms. Answer: 706

Over Supination Syndrome

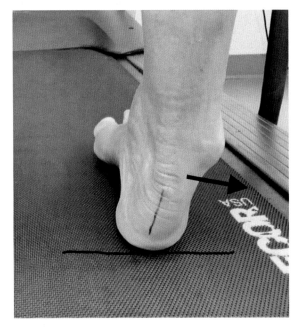

Supination during the contact phase of gait is abnormal

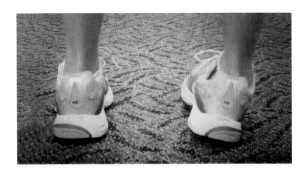

Simple image of abnormal supination causing lateral instability and possible ankle sprain

Now let's talk about contact phase oversupination, and why I think it is so much worse than most cases I see of pronation (with hundreds of exceptions). When the foot strikes the ground, the entire limb above it is internally rotating, and so must the foot for all to go well. Supination of the foot, or external foot rotation, at a time when the limb is internally rotating, will produce a strain somewhere from the foot, ankle and up the leg. Also, by replacing the mechanism for shock absorption in pronation, you now have a petri dish for stress fractures, joint arthralgias, and low back pain. Finally, contact phase supination causes, and is sometimes called, lateral instability. Do not take this lightly? Whenever the word instability is used in the lower extremity, weight bearing will be affected, falls will occur at a higher rate, and our job of rehabilitation becomes more challenging. A little over supination, Dr. Root defined the tipping point as 3 degrees past neutral subtalar joint, and most say 3 degrees past vertical. Simply ⅛ to ¼ inch valgus wedges can help. There is no over the counter insert for supinators that I have any experience with, but some low arched inserts with a deep heel cup can be a starting point.

Here is the list I give to students on the injuries created by excessive supination, which is also called under pronation, and also called lateral instability. Someone may be an excess supinator only when they wear certain shoes. Someone may be structured to overly supinate even barefoot. Excessive supination causes injuries because of lateral instability, because the lack of pronation means no shock absorption, because there is lateral weight bearing on the foot for a prolonged time, and there is excessive medial loading of the ankle and knee. Injuries can also occur since there is knee extension at contact, not the normal knee flexion. Here is a summary of the problems related to oversupination. These injuries include:

1. Hammertoes
2. Lateral Metatarsalgia
3. Tailor's Bunion
4. 4th and/or 5th metatarsal fractures
5. Cuboid pain
6. Lateral Ankle Instability
7. Peroneal Strain
8. Haglund's Deformity
9. Medial Ankle Impingement
10. Fibular Stress Fractures
11. Proximal Tib-Fib Sprain
12. Medial Knee Compartment
13. Knee Arthralgias
14. Lateral Collateral Ligament Sprain (Knee)
15. Lateral Hamstring Strain
16. Iliotibial Band Syndrome
17. Femoral Stress Fractures
18. Hip Arthralgias
19. Sacroiliac Inflammation
20. Low Back Pain

Hammertoes due to the lateral foot and ankle instability can be caused by over supination. Abnormal supination is the most unstable situation the foot has to try to stabilize. A common way to attempt more foot stability is by clawing of the toes, which can then lead to hammertoe deformities. In fact, when a patient says out of the blue that they noticed one or both feet were developing hammertoes, I immediately try to see if there is instability causing it. High arched feet with a normal increased metatarsal declination are already prone to hammertoe development. If you add supination instability to a high arched foot, the chance of development of hammertoes is around 100%. A recent

patient reminded me of this instability issue and to look for any source. For her, the instability was caused by double vision from complications of a recent cataract procedure. Therefore, a patient can be unstable from many sources leading to the gradual development of hammertoes as clenching of the toes initially seems to anchor the toes down better. As the toes come off the ground completely, they are useless in any attempt at foot stability.

Lateral metatarsalgia is a common problem related to over supination. This abnormal supination typically occurs in the contact phase of gait, but can linger throughout midstance into propulsion. This abnormal subtalar joint supination causes an overload of the lateral forefoot with lateral metatarsalgia symptoms developing. The treatment can be complicated since orthotic corrections for this lateral overload sometimes require the most corrective force be placed on the sore area (like in cases of everted forefoot deformities that need to be balanced in orthotic devices), however there are many modifications to attempt to off weight the sore area and increase weight behind it, in front of it, or both. Goal: if you have to compromise support, make sure that the patient is still stable.

Practical Biomechanics Question #483: Lateral support in custom orthotic devices utilizing Root techniques comes from balancing forefoot valgus situations. What are the 3 common everted forefoot deformities that can lead to lateral foot overload and one main tibial problem producing the same lateral overload? A: 707

Tailor's bunion development and resultant pain is caused by both overpronation in patients with a high degree for forefoot abduction on the rearfoot, or excessive supination with excess lateral loading of the foot. Tailor's bunions on the fifth metatarsal head are so much less problematic as the same degree of deformity in first metatarsal bunions. One of the causes of tailors bunions is this lateral forefoot overload due to excessive supination which produces a chronic subluxation on the cuboid-fifth metatarsal joint articulation. The fifth ray motion when overloaded plantarly is towards eversion, abduction, and dorsiflexion. The abduction of the 5th metatarsal leads to a widening of the 5th ray away from the 4th ray, and obvious appearance of the tailor's bunion.

4th and/or 5th metatarsal fractures occur with oversupination forces in athletics, or bone weakened patients. This excessive supination causes lateral overload of the 4th and 5th metatarsals which both articulate with the cuboid. When that overload is fairly rapid, like in training too quickly for a marathon, either the 4th metatarsal or the 5th metatarsal may develop a stress fracture. Which metatarsal breaks depends on the ability of these 2 metatarsals to move superiorly in reaction to the ground forces. They will always move differently and sometimes the fifth metatarsal moves upward enough that the fourth metatarsal takes the weight. Typically, most patients I have seen have a slight plantar flexed fifth metatarsal that takes the excessive weight and develops stress fractures, like a Jones fracture. Angle

of gait issues also affect how weight is transferred through the foot during stance. A more internal angle of gait, even without supination tendencies, can hold weight more lateral for a longer period of time throughout the stance phase. In a dropped metatarsal arch, or a super unstable 5th ray, all the weight goes to the 4th metatarsal head.

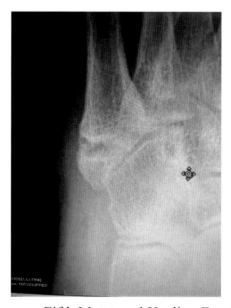

Fifth Metatarsal Healing Fracture

Practical Biomechanics Question #484: If excessive supination will shift weight more lateral in a foot, what are some reasons that the 4th metatarsal develops the overuse injury, not the 5th? Answer: 707

Cuboid pain from overload can be caused by over supination. This excessive supination causes lateral overload on the cuboid and then some form of joint dysfunction and ensuing pain. The cuboid just after heel contact is acted upon by the powerful gastroc-soleus complex. This complex contracts to push the cuboid towards the supporting surface. This produces a very stable midfoot and a key element in re-supination of the foot. With over supination, that cuboid loading goes too far, and depending what ligaments are loose, the cuboid is dorsiflexed possibly across various joints: calcaneocuboid, cuboid-third cuneiform, cuboid-4th or 5th metatarsals, or cuboid-navicular. This is opposite of cuboid syndrome post inversion ankle sprain where the cuboid gets stuck plantarly. The famous cuboid whip is designed to dorsiflex (or superiorly translate) the cuboid when stuck below its normal position.

Practical Biomechanics Question #485: Cuboid pain can be produced by lateral overload. What 5 joint articulations could be involved? Answer: 707

    Lateral ankle instability is a common problem, especially inversion ankle sprain causing excessive supination. This excessive supination at contact phase is also called lateral instability. It is a disastrous motion that when it occurs will rob the foot of shock absorption (as it should be pronating), and places an extension force on the knee when it should be flexing. Yet, it is the lateral stress at the ankle that can cause some of the most troublesome issues. When you combine this lateral foot and ankle instability with an unstable shoe or terrain or old sprains, the patient may be set up for chronic issues. Sometimes, it is hard to discover the chicken or the egg. Lateral ankle instability is brought on by injuries produced by the subtalar supination, or the instability itself (from a previous injury or ligamentous laxity) can cause excessive

supination. The pain from lateral ankle instability then can be acute when a new injury occurs, or chronic in all the areas excessive supination causes pain even the lateral or medial ankle areas, etc.

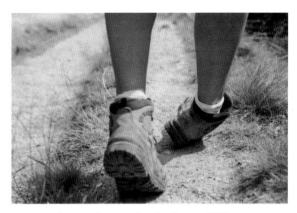

Inversion twist during a Hike

Practical Biomechanics Question #486: How can lateral ankle instability produced by over supination can medial ankle pain? Why in an acute inversion sprain is pain medially possibly indicative of something significant? Answer: 707

    Peroneal strain is caused by excessive supination. This excessive subtalar joint supination stresses the lateral side of the foot and ankle, and one of the ways the body tries to protect itself is by excessively contracting the peroneal tendons. It can be both the peroneus longus or the peroneus brevis, or more one than the other. It may be that the peroneal tendons are weak anyway, and can not react well when the foot is in an unstable lateral position or motion. Like the complexity of the posterior tibial, or all of the extrinsic ankle muscles, straining the peroneals can give you pain from its origin on the fibula to the insertions on the first (peroneus longus) or fifth (peroneus brevis) metatarsals, or anywhere in between. I warn patients who have pain around the lateral malleolus, and get an MRI for some reason, that the tendons can look torn on MRI and be totally strong and non painful in examination. This is a problem with the way the peroneal tendon turns around the corner of the ankle onto the foot, and the MRI slice looks like they are torn when not. Also many peroneal tendons normally have multiple fibers that look like micro-tearing. Practical Biomechanics Question #487: How do you separately muscle test the peroneus brevis to peroneus longus?

Haglund's deformity and pain is caused by excessive supination. The posterior superior lateral corner of the calcaneus is closer to the heel counter of shoes than the medial corner, and therefore will take more friction or stress from that interaction. Excessive supination at heel contact will magnify that lateral pressure on the posterior corner. Correction of the lateral rotation of excessive supination does 2 very positive things to the Haglund's bump aka retrocalcaneal exostosis or pump bump. The first function of an orthotic device is in minimizing the lateral drift of the heel therefore decreasing the force that creates or irritates the deformity. The second function of the orthotic device is in simply raising the heel slightly so that there is less pressure in the same area.

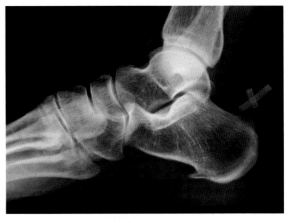

Haglunds at the posterior superior and lateral corner of the heel bone (under the X)

Medial ankle impingement is a very common problem related to excessive supination. This excessive supination affects the talus by moving it medially within the ankle mortise to crowd the medial talar dome and medial talar border on the lateral surface of the medial malleolus. If that inversion is sudden, like in an inversion ankle sprain, bony injury can occur to the talus or tibia. If the inversion is less forceful, but consistent, as in activities of repetitive motion like walking, hiking, biking, etc, the soft tissue can get irritated. When I make orthotics for patients, Inverted type in particular, but even Root Balanced, I can create an excessive inversion force that leads to medial ankle impingement. It is very common that the patient is fine until the shoe starts to break down laterally increasing the inversion force across all joints. This is one of the reasons you follow up your orthotic care with visits every 6-9 months after dispense.

Practical Biomechanics Question #487: With the high cost of athletic shoes, patients can be prone to wearing them too long.

When they begin to break down laterally, even in a patient with normal biomechanics, what types of ankle problems can they develop related to over supination? A: 707

Fibular stress fractures are a great example of over supination. This excessive subtalar joint supination increases lateral weight bearing in the foot, but that weight bearing stress goes medially into the talus and tibia as just described, and not the fibula. The excessive supination affects the fibula by producing an unstable lateral ankle which compensates with tremendous muscle pull of the peroneals. The pull can be so stressful that it breaks the fibula by muscle contraction only. I once treated a semi-professional ballet dancer that sickled (excessive supination in ballet terms) en pointe. The teacher had been trying to correct this technique error, but she broke her fibula 3 different times in the course of 2 years. Finally, both better technique and a thin sewn thread along the lateral border of the end of her pointe shoe fixed the problem.

Practical Biomechanics Question #488: So many stress fractures (or full fractures) can occur by abnormal muscle contraction only. If a patient presents with lateral leg pain, why would it be important to differentiate the pain from bone pain versus peroneal muscle or tendon pain?

Proximal tib-fib sprain can be caused by excessive supination. Excessive supination increases the medial weight bearing across the knee joint and opens up the lateral knee joint capsule. This can be used to our advantage in cases of lateral meniscal tears or compression syndrome, either post operatively to decompress the lateral compartment, or in an attempt to avoid surgery in non-bucket handle tears, by adding varus wedges or inversion forces into custom orthotic devices. However, in opening up the lateral capsule of the knee, you may also cause instability at the proximal tib-fib joint which can get grade 1 sprain symptoms. It is important to follow up on these cases and check for improvements and any new symptoms.

Practical Biomechanics Question #489: What 2 very important structures attach into the head of the fibula? Answer: 707

Practical Biomechanics Question #490: How could over tightness of the lateral hamstring lead to proximal tib-fib symptoms? Answer: 707

Medial knee compartment overload can occur with excessive supination by overloading the medial knee joint. Medial knee meniscus problems and degenerative joint problems plague society. It is somewhat a problem of knee extension, whereas societies that bend their knees more get lateral meniscus issues. The patient presents with pain, and sometimes swelling, along the medial knee joint line. This one problem is why over supination has to be more addressed in society. In school, over 40 years ago, I was taught if a patient with new orthotic devices complained of medial knee pain, that I had over supinated them.

Practical Biomechanics Question #491: What side of the knee is compressed when you supinate the foot? Answer: 708

Knee arthralgias can be produced by excessive supination forces. Excessive supination jars the knees by robbing the foot of its shock absorption issues. Correcting the supination can soften the knees at impact, even when using a plastic device. Since deep knee pain can present in various ways, and sometimes very hard to localize, it may be the medial knee compartment overload syndrome when over supination is noted in gait. This same abnormal supination which places a varus stress at the knee, also causes an extension motion across the knee. The more extended a knee joint is, the more potential of compression force.

Lateral Knee collateral ligament sprain can be caused by excessive supination. This excessive supination opens the lateral knee joint line and can sprain the lateral collateral ligament attaching into the head of the fibula.

Lateral hamstring strain can be caused by over supination. This excessive supination opens up the lateral joint line being protected by the lateral hamstrings attaching into the head of the fibula. The lateral hamstrings may be strained for this function. The hamstrings themselves are knee joint flexors, whereas excessive supination puts an extension force on the knee when it should be flexing. This may also strain the hamstrings. With this extension force at the knee, there can be more jarring/compression. The hamstrings may strain in an attempt to flex the knee thereby relaxing the tension within the knee joint itself.

Iliotibial band syndrome can be caused by either over pronation or over supination. This excessive supination of the foot causes lateral instability affecting the soft tissues that guard the whole lateral one half of our extremities. I have talked about the effect on the peroneal tendons and hamstrings, but the iliotibial band is probably the most affected above the ankle with over supination. The iliotibial band functions to protect the lateral side of the hip and the lateral side of the knee at foot strike. It is a common running injury since the force that needs to be stabilized can be 7 times that of walking, and running mechanics tend naturally to be more inverted for longer times. Excessive supination of the foot on top of all these other factors can easily lead to an overload of the iliotibial band as it tries to protect the hip and knee.

Practical Biomechanics Question #492: Would a patient with a higher than normal Q Angle be more likely to get iliotibial band syndrome while running? Answer: 708

Femoral stress fractures can be caused by over supination. This excessive supination robs the body of its foot shock absorption leading to increased stress up the leg. Excessive supination also causes knee extension at foot strike accentuating jarring forces at the knee and hip. Femoral stress fractures in relatively young patients is seen in runners where the athlete has to absorb up to 7 times body weight while downhill running. If you add low Vitamin D, inadequate diet issues, shoes that have broken down recently, or some combination of factors, and a tendency to supinate, it is easy to imagine the femur developing stress reactions and fractures.

Practical Biomechanics Question #493: For shock absorption problems in the lower leg, the Hannaford custom orthotic device, primarily discussed in the next book, is ideal. What is the type of material a Hannaford is made out of, and can you also correct for pronation or supination? A:708

Hip arthralgias can be caused by excessive supination. This excessive supination robs the body of needed shock absorption and can cause increased joint loading at the knee, hip, and sacroiliac joints.

Sacroiliac joint inflammation from upward jamming of the joint can be caused by over supination. The sacroiliac joint is a gliding joint that primarily moves in the sagittal plane both inferiorly and superiorly. When the heel contacts the ground and the knee is straight, that force created can drive up the ilium on the stationary sacrum. The SI joint is said to be stuck superiorly and symptoms can occur. If you have ever misjudged the height of a step and landed with a jerk, the sacroiliac joint takes that force and can be placed in a wrong position causing joint symptoms, often mistaken as hip or back pain. Excessive subtalar joint supination extends the knee and can force this scenario more insidiously from

repetitive motion. The patient is then unaware of a cause but complains of chronic back pain.

Practical Biomechanics Question #494: As the SI joint moves inferiorly, it also moves in what direction? When palpating the ASIS during lower extremity limb length exam, if you find the right ASIS to be forward to the left, what does that mean? Answer: 708

Low back pain from poor shock absorption or excessive hamstring pull is common with excessive foot supination at heel contact. We know that our hamstrings are tighter when we straighten the knee, and looser when we bend our knee. As we straighten the knee from excessive supination, this puts more of a stretch on the hamstrings and gastrocnemius that both cross the back of the knee joint. The hamstrings attach into the ischial tuberosities (sit bones). This tension in the hamstrings pulls down on the pelvis to extend the hip at a time in gait (contact phase) when the hip should be flexing. This extension force on the hip and pelvis also straightens our back causing muscle and disc irritations.

Now that we have gone through many of the problems related to over pronation and over supination, you will first spot these patterns in your historical examination. It is tempting to ask the patient why they are here today, identify that problem, and begin treatment. However, past problems, and other less troublesome issues that they do not want to bother you with, are very important to know about with respect to getting to a reversible cause and treatment. For example, a patient presents with posterior tibial pain acutely, but also has nagging medial shin splints and iliotibial band issues. These can all be tied to overpronation. This patient also has a history of plantar fasciitis, some sort of lateral midfoot problem, and some low back pain. Now, we have 6 past and present problems related to overpronation in a runner during the last two years. I propose this is a different athlete than one with a one week history of posterior tibial pain and no past history of problems. The history here highlights more of an importance to correct the pronation for good with state of the art orthotic devices, stable running shoes, and physical therapy to learn how to appropriately strengthen and stretch. We are on the patient's side, we have recognized a repeatable pattern, and how we have to protect them so that they can keep going for years in whatever their sport or activity.

Treatment of overpronation or oversupination has been both previously mentioned and part of the chapter ahead on components of custom made functional foot orthotics (Chapter 13 of Book 4). I suggest that anyone skilled in the treatment of the pronation and supination spectrum from severe supination to severe pronation should be able to have their orthotic laboratory the following 6 prescriptions:

1. Severe Supination
2. Moderate Supination
3. Mild Supination
4. Vertical (Neutral in the Ideal Foot)
5. Mild Pronation
6. Moderate Pronation
7. Severe Pronation

As the orthotic laboratory is manufacturing your orthotic prescription, you are getting the patients into shoes that match their pronator or supinator needs. This can be harder for supinators, where at the severe level can even need midsole or outsole wedging to help. You can also send them for 3 physical therapy sessions to learn how to stretch and strengthen the appropriate muscles. The appropriate muscles in general to be strengthened for pronators are:

- Foot Intrinsics
- Posterior Tibial
- Anterior Tibial
- Peroneus Longus
- Gastrocnemius and Soleus
- Lateral Hamstring
- Sartorius
- Piriformis
- Gluteus Medius
- Iliopsoas

The appropriate muscles in general to be strengthened for supinators are:

- Foot Intrinsics
- Peroneus Longus and Brevis
- Medial Hamstrings
- Hip Internal Rotators
- Hip Adductors

You have to also remove equinus forces with pronators by stretching out the achilles and medial hamstrings, if and only if they are tight. You have to stretch the lateral hamstrings and hip abductors, including the Iliotibial band, if they are tight.

Practical Biomechanics Question #495: What are the seven Rxs for orthotic laboratories based on the pronation to supination spectrum? Answer: 708

Chapter 10: Limb Length Discrepancy

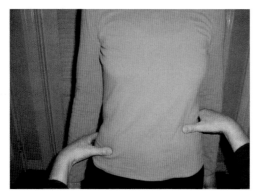

Standing Landmarks are Used to Check for Possible Leg Length Discrepancies

Introduction

Limb length discrepancy, also known as short leg syndrome or leg length difference, occurs in a structural, functional, or combination state. From a biomechanical standpoint, it means that the hip heights are not equal causing the right and left sides of the body to function asymmetrical (structural), or caused by the right and left sides of the body functioning asymmetrical (functional). For day to day activities, the symptoms of leg length discrepancy may not show up until one is in their 60s or later, but from a sports standpoint, a slight difference in the leg length over 3000 miles of running or cycling or rowing, for example, can be devastating and affect the athlete at an early age. When the hips are unequal (structural or functional) which leans the body to one side (called limb dominance), the body will compensate with every motion to keep the eyes level to the ground. In fact, we are so good at compensating in life, that patients are surprised when I tell them they have a ½ inch short leg when they are 70 years old. And, of course, this is combined with chronic low back pain for starters, which may be why they came into your office in the first place. Definitely the older one gets, the harder it is to adapt to structural deviations or to changes in biomechanics, so starting lift therapy for a running achilles injury in their 30s can help or prevent their low back problem in their 70s and 80s. It is up to the practitioner to emphasize that even keeping a one half correction (50%) in a permanent treatment is very preventative for the future.

The 3 types of limb length discrepancy that a patient may have are pure structural, pure functional, and a combination of some structural and some functional. Measurement presented here is osteopathic, with tape measurements proven unreliable to the author. The best time to measure for leg length is when the patient has their custom orthotic devices already designed to eliminate functional variations of foot pronation. A one degree change in resting heel position between feet can be a one sixteenth inch difference in drop of the hips. The best clinical approach is to palpate the hip heights standing barefoot, build up under the short leg by 3 mm lift material incrementally (I use sheets of 3 mm top cover I have in my office) until the hips are even, thus declaring the working limb length calculation. Remeasuring later with any functional change occurs like adding varus wedges or custom made orthotic devices, or postoperative any foot and ankle surgery, may change the amount of lift needed. This is also important after any severe lower extremity injury or surgery, including knee or hip replacements. After I measure limb length standing, I do like to look for foot asymmetries immediately that could be in play. If you just imagine the 2 scenarios: long leg measured on the side of more pronation (meaning if that pronation was fixed the side would even be longer), and long leg on the opposite side of the more pronated foot (meaning if you correct the pronation unevenness the long leg may not be long any more). I think it is good to take the approach that every patient with a leg length difference is probably a combination type: some structural and some functional, so you are not declaring the leg length measurement you got is carved in stone.

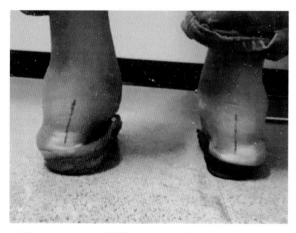

The 8 degree difference in foot pronation measured by RCSP on the current orthotic devices means functionally the left side is one-half inch shorter or 8/16 inch. If a new orthotic device leveled the heels to both verticals, the lift being used would have to be adjusted.

Another problem is that the measurements are hard to standardize with each discipline adding their own rules. I will tell you what has worked for me over the years and that has helped so many patients. I use the profession of osteopathic medicine to guide my practice of lift therapy, although I am not sure how far I have changed my general rules since I began to treat leg length differences in 1979.

Short leg syndrome can account for a huge amount of problems, and probably one of the biggest is chronic low back pain, yet it is typically ignored by the medical profession. If it is addressed at all, the treatment can be just with heel lifts, sometimes only attached to orthotics, and often not high enough, or on the wrong side. There is also a psychological stigma to the patient when you want to put the lift on the outside of the shoe for the best stability.

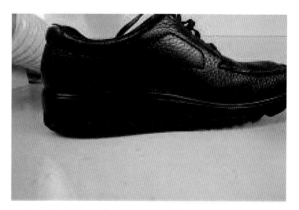

One half inch outsole lift used for Short Leg Syndrome

Historical Review and Gait Evaluation Findings

Even in the historical review, as we begin to ask the patient questions regarding their current injury and past injuries or painful areas, patterns may be seen of a consistent injury history on the same side through the years. This however can be skewed due to other past injuries affecting either leg like an ACL tear having nothing to do with limb length difference, and the dominance of their right or left handedness. From a podiatrist standpoint, and at least what I can offer to the patient, a history of low back or hip pain with walking or exercise, may be related to the unevenness at the spine and pelvis created by a short leg. This is less clear if their hip or low back pain mainly occurs while sleeping or sitting. This is very important when you talk to any patient about their low back pain in terms of when it occurs. If their pain is primarily related to walking or standing, then there could be a significant solution with lift and stretching protocols (especially the hamstrings). If their pain is primarily related to sitting or sleeping, there is less of a strong association with short leg syndrome (although still may be present). Therefore, the 3 common times the low back primarily presents:

- Standing or Walking--strong association with LLD
- Sitting
- Sleeping or Lying

Yet, limb length discrepancy may never present with back or hip pain, but a long history of same sided complaints (left iliotibial band, left shoulder, left upper pain, left knee) spreading over the course of 20 years.

As I discussed in chapter 3 (Book 1), gait evaluation is one of the most common point in our clinic time that we begin to suspect a limb length discrepancy exists. The common signs noted in gait are dominance to one side, varying arm swing patterns, shoulder drop, head tilt to one side, higher belt line on one side, asymmetry in hip motion (seen at the knees), in fact asymmetry in most observed lower extremity motions. There is a summary of the gait findings in limb length difference:

- Dominance (Lean) to One Side
- Varying Arm Swing Patterns
- Shoulder Drop
- Head Tilt to One Side
- Higher Belt to One Side
- Asymmetrical Hip Motion
- Asymmetrical Lower Extremity Motion

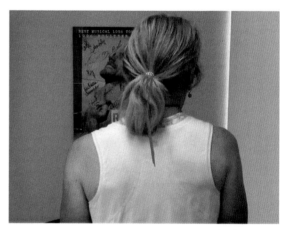

Head Tilt to the Short Leg (classic presentation)

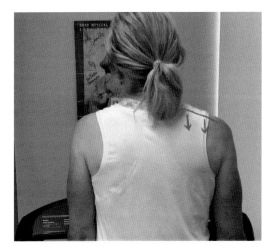

Shoulder Drop to the Long Side (classic presentation)

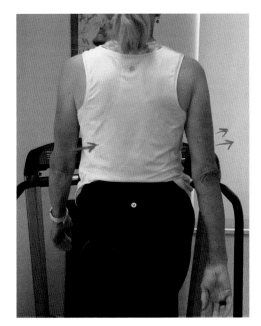

Asymmetrical Arm Swing demonstrates further away from body non-dominant side

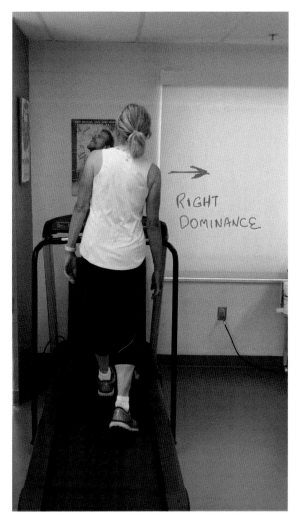

Dominance to One Side typically to the Longer Side

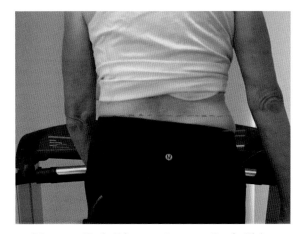

Uneven Belt Line on Longer Left Side

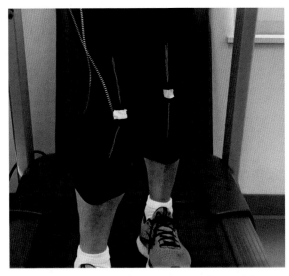

Asymmetrical Hip Motion reflected by Knee Excursion with more Internal Knee Position on more Pronating Side

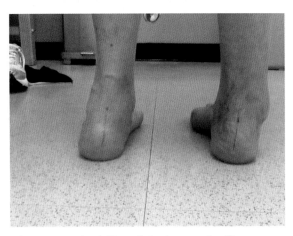

Asymmetrical Foot Motion typically more pronation on the longer side

Practical Biomechanics Question #496: What are 7 common gait signs of a leg length difference? Answer: 708

General Rules About Lift Therapy and Measurements

Before I get further into the discussion, I do want to give you my general rules. The rules that I follow are:

- Full length lifts are preferable to heel lifts (further discussion soon)

Practical Biomechanics Question #497: Explain why a runner with a short leg would do better with a full length lift versus a heel lift while running hills. Answer: 708

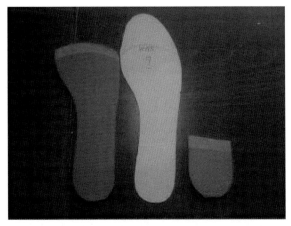

Typically Full Length Lifts are to the Sulcus eliminating too much digital pressure

- The measurement of leg length shortness can be totally different if you use osteopathic versus chiropractic rules since their reference points are different, with osteopathic used here documented close to bony measurements
- The mantra of treatment is "Start Low and Go Slow".
- Until you have fully analyzed the effects of orthotic devices versus short leg lifts on a patient, keep the

two treatments separate, when both are being deployed.

- If you first evaluate a patient and feel that their symptoms will require lifts and orthotic devices, start the lift therapy at the first visit while you are waiting for the manufacturing of the custom orthotic devices.
- Most athletic shoes can take up to 3/8th inch (10 mm) lift material as an internal lift under the shoe insert or an orthotic device.
- Treatment is classically half the measured height, but this must be followed by symptom response. Some symptoms require full correction at least temporarily before you attempt to back the correction down some.
- Outsole or midsole lifting is usually after some insole lifting has helped symptoms, and is started on one pair of shoes the patient uses often
- Outsole or midsole lifting tends to be full height under the heel, tapered as you go forward, to one half thickness at the metatarsals and then quickly tapered at the toes. This has to be modified if the patient feels that they are falling forward or being blocked from rolling forward.
- When using outsole or midsole lifts, they produce a slightly greater change to the body than just internal shoe lifts (softer). This is due to the greater density of the more durable external shoe lift. When a patient feels comfortable with ⅜ inch internal lifting, I typically start at ¼

inch external shoe lifting due to this effect.

- When using outsole or midsole lifts, care should be taken to build in some flexibility under the ball of the foot. You can see from the photo of the external lift below that cuts are made from medial to lateral to increase the flexibility. Cobblers can punch holes into the ball of the foot area of the lift material to keep flexibility. Unless there is a reason for forefoot rigidity, you have to emphasize that you want the finished product to still be flexible.

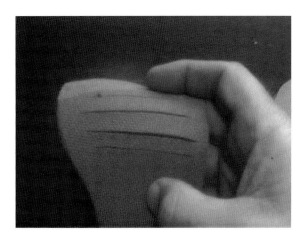

- Lifts, in general, force the ground further away from the foot, and at times cause tripping (with some increase in the elderly population). Elderly patients tend to need the lifts the most, but have to be treated with much more care, and with a lot more compromise.
- Any additional lift added to the treatment must be accompanied with gait evaluation to check that the patient looks and feels more stable (even going from ⅛ to ¼ inch lift)

Practical Biomechanics Question #498: If a patient has chronic low back pain for years, and you have measured around one half inch short right side, how would you get them into lift therapy smartly? Answer 708

When I watch any patient walk, or perform their activities, I watch for the smooth symmetry of motion. When the gait or technique should be symmetrical, but is not, and I observe some of the following: dominance to one side, asymmetrical arm swing, uneven shoulders and beltline, and asymmetrical foot function, I begin to think about the possibility of leg length difference. Then I palpate the evenness of the anterior superior iliac crests, the iliac crests, and the greater trochanters of the femur.

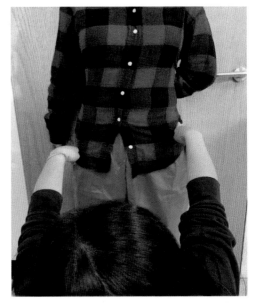

Palpation for level Greater Trochanters

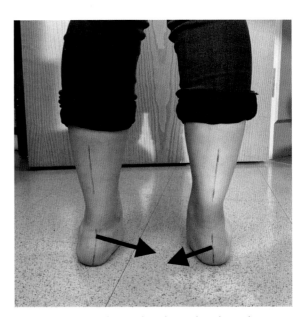

When you evaluate leg length, also observe foot asymmetry which could be involved with the more pronated side dropping the pelvis on that side

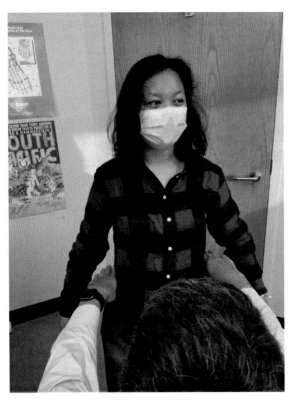

Palpation Iliac Crests with Hands Parallel and Examiner's Eyes at Level of Exam

If I want to work on pelvic tilts, I will also check the posterior superior iliac spines. I work hard to keep my hands or fingers parallel and on the same spots right to left. If all 3 landmarks show that one side is low,

I feel safe calling it a short leg (and assume it is a combination of structural shortness somewhere and functional component like unequal pronation). I can try to just estimate which is the shorter side if this is during a cursory examination (and just start with a 3 mm lift anyway). I can begin a more detailed examination by building up under the apparent short leg (using material about 3 mm thickness as separate lifts in my office) until the hips are level (I would still start with 3 mm no matter what I measured). I may take a Standing AP Pelvis X-ray barefoot in normal stance if the examination is confusing, or the patient is obese, or there are conflicting measurements in the past, or if the pain is so chronic that the findings are crucial to be corrected now!!

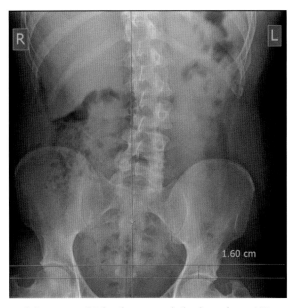

16 mm or ⅝ inch on weight bearing AP Pelvic Standing X Ray barefoot in normal stance

Biomechanics of Heel Lifts

Since the general rule of treating leg length discrepancy is with heel lifts, and commonly heel lifts permanently attached to custom made foot orthotic devices, I must discuss the many advantages of heel lifts and some blatant disadvantages. The biomechanics of placing a heel lift into a shoe for the correction of a short leg is quite interesting. For any individual patient, the pros or cons of wearing the lift can win out. And for any patient, this can vary from shoe to shoe. So, why I prefer a full length lift overall, I will question the hundreds of my patients on the success or failure of previously applied heel lifts. Heel lifts increase the tone in the achilles by slightly activating the calf making it easier to move forward. Heel lifts lift you up in the shoe adding to some instability at times since the heel counter does not grab your foot as much, and also allows the patient to clear a sore spot (like in Haglund's heel bump). Heel lifts do nothing to the limb length correction anytime the patient is on the ball of the foot (as running up a hill). Heel lifts are better than full length lifts for actual fit in a shoe. Heel lifts can stress the midfoot, where there is no support if the patient is not using an orthotic device at the same time, especially when the lift gets over ¼ inch. In contrast to full length lifts, heel lifts do not push the patient's shoe away from the foot at push off, adding to tripping problems. In summary, these are some of my perceived differences between heel lifts and full length lifts, that must be individualized for each patient and for each shoe:

- Heel lifts increase calf/achilles tone
- Heel lifts make the shoe less stable
- Heel lifts crowd the shoe less
- Heel lifts can help Haglund's deformity pain
- Heel lifts do not help when the weight is on the metatarsals
- Heel lifts are simpler to use
- Heel lifts do not push the shoe away from the foot at push off causing tripping
- Heel lifts can make a patient feel like they are falling forward
- Heel lifts can strain the forefoot due to increase pressure from being tilted forward
- Heel lifts can strain the midfoot due to lack of support (suspended in the air)

I have seen both successes and failures with heel lifts and full length lifts. There are so many factors involved, and I usually end up using full length lifts sometimes and heel lifts at other times in the same patient.

Practical Biomechanics Question #499: There are pros and cons with using heel lifts vs full length lifts. What would the obvious choice be in a runner? Answer: 708

Common Symptoms of Leg Length Difference

Besides seeing obvious gait changes of leg length difference, I have a small list of patient diagnoses that I always want to know if one leg is shorter. These areas are:
- Low Back Pain
- Hip Pain
- Lower Extremity nerves problems: Morton's Neuroma, Tarsal Tunnel, etc.
- Iliotibial Band Syndrome
- Unilateral Achilles Problems
- Pronatory Problems with Unilateral Pronation (typically long leg)

The pelvis sits at the base of our spines, and if the pelvis is tilted, the spine becomes tilted. There are various stresses that buildup in our spines, pelvis, and hips. Most hip pain is on the longer side in general. Therefore, one of the top treatments Podiatrists can do for pain in this area of the body when there is a leg length difference, is to use lift therapy. It is so effective, and so under utilized, I have to wonder if so many more patients preventatively starting using lift therapy in their 30s what would happen as they age. These uneven tilts with a tendency to lean to one side of the body can cause a myriad of muscle compensations to attempt to right the ship. I have seen so many cases of iliotibial band or peroneal strain resolved with lift therapy. I imagine that they were working overtime to right the ship or the leaning tower of Pisa.

Uneven tilts are only one aspect that causes problems from the back down, or the back up. Compensatory supination of the short leg or over pronation of the long leg can create supinatory or pronatory problems just elaborately discussed in Chapter 9. We can understand compensating for a long leg by pronating more to flatten the arch on the long side, in order to make the leg less long. This process of pronation works with gravity and little muscle activity to compensate this way for a long leg. But the compensation for a short leg, to raise the arch, to fight against gravity, is a difficult task. Unilateral early heel lift on the short side leading to achilles strain is one example that tends to fit this model. And, we know that some feet just supinate more easily than others like forefoot valgus feet versus forefoot varus feet.

Back in Book 1 I discussed that our treatment of patients has to involve all 3 sources of pain: mechanical, inflammatory, and neuropathic. Patients present routinely with neuropathic pain symptoms, sometimes vague, sometimes more obvious, in the lower extremity. I also discussed how all three types of pain could be treated in all three ways: mechanical treatments, inflammatory treatments, and neuropathic treatments. One of the ways we can definitely help nerve pain or symptoms in the lower extremity is to mechanically level the base of the spine with our lift therapy. So, patients presenting with any nerve symptoms like Tarsal Tunnel, Morton's Neuroma, etc, with a short leg, should be started on lift therapy.

Treatment of Leg Length

When I measure limb length in a patient, no matter what the initial measurement, I tell the patient that the numbers are only accurate 80% of the time (that is, 20% of the time the short leg may actually be the other side or there could be no shortness at all or measurement off by a few millimeters). I then watch them walk in ¼ or ⅜ inch lifts on the short side under their insert or orthotic device. If the dominance I saw on one side, usually the longer leg in

adults (also 80%), disappears and the patient can usually feel an improvement in stability, I typically feel that I am going in the right direction. For some of the reasons I shared above, I may get an AP Pelvic Standing X-ray barefoot in a normal stance to document my findings. However, any asymmetry of foot position, with one arch lower than the other, will put a functional component into the x ray with the more pronated foot lowering the hip height. When the longer leg pronates more than the shorter leg, it begins to even out the difference. When the shorter leg pronates more, since there can be two separate biomechanical faults acting at the same time, it will make that side even shorter at the hip on x-ray. Therefore, if there is asymmetrical pronation, before you x ray, attempt to correct that asymmetry with orthotic devices, or wait 6 months for the lifts to affect the numbers. By this I mean, if the patient only pronated because of the long leg, and you use lifts to correct for the long leg, the pronation should resolve in 6 months.

Practical Biomechanics Question #500: When one side is more pronated, orthotic Rxs can be to correct for the asymmetry or avoid it. If a long leg pronates more, and the orthotic correction is more support on that side, what is this doing to the asymmetry of the long leg? Answer: 708

So, **Decision #1**, I make a decision on what side is short, then decide if it is urgent to x-ray or wait (only 20% of my patients will ever get this x-ray). I then decide (**Decision #2**) if orthotic devices due to the rearfoot asymmetrical motion are needed initially, or only after lift therapy is completed and evaluated for stability and symptom response. **Decision #3**, I then start on lifts. The lifts are typically ⅛ inch to the sulcus (so the toes have room) for 2 weeks, and then another slightly shorter sulcus length lift for another 2 weeks. This is when I want to see the patient back. Any new pain or feeling of instability or that something is not right when they go up in the lifts means they take the new lift out until I see them. I always have the patient leave the office with a good feeling with the ⅛ inch on the day we start lift therapy. This is how I will start for leg length ¼ inch or higher in all cases.

Typically, if I measure that they are ½ inch short or so, on the first visit I want to watch them walk with their full correction to see if it changed their limb dominance. Limb dominance is seen as little as ⅛ inch, but in all cases of ¼ inch and higher. The patient, not being used to this amount, will feel weird and I warn them of that. I tell them that I want to see a reduction or elimination of limb dominance (them leaning), and I also palpate the same landmarks to look and see if it is equal or more equal than without lifts. They will typically leave my office with (3) one eighth inch lifts to get used sulcus length, and one ⅛ and one ¼ inch heel lift. The heel lifts will be used when the second or third sulcus length lift crowds the toes too much, or in shoes that can only take heel lifts. I need the patient to get used to the lifts in any form possible.

Any activity that has a huge component of repetitive stress seems to do well with lifts. I am excited about pressure sensors in shoes that will document the abnormal asymmetrical loading of the long and short leg in runners, rowing, cyclists, etc. However, I love to place some leather over any insert that goes into a shoe when I have some in stock. You can very quickly see the asymmetrical weight distribution at the heel (with one side, typically the long side) loading with more pressure.

Any time we talk about asymmetry you have to mention our natural asymmetrical motion due to being right or left handed. The general lower extremity implications if we are right handed is that the right side is our movement side and our left side is our support side. And, of course, the opposite if you are left handed. Therefore, when I watch someone walk up and down my clinic halls, I can typically pick out if they are right or left handed (with only the lefties being impressed with my observation). If you watch a right handed patient, they are more stable on the left side and there is more mobility on the right side (as they are unconsciously preparing to plant their left foot and hit the ball with their right foot). I bring this up because some people are really right or left handed, and this lack of ambidexterity solidifies a certain neuro-muscular rigidity. They look very asymmetrical and they function that way. You can be misled into thinking the asymmetry is related to a short leg issue.

Practical Biomechanics Question #501: If a patient is walking, and their left side is more unstable than their right, and they are left handed, what could that mean (many answers)? Answer: 709

Common Examples

One of the classic examples I teach to my students involves a lesson I learned early in my practice. I worked with another podiatrist who had properly diagnosed that the short right leg was causing some right sided (uni-lateral) achilles tendonitis. He gave the athlete a standard heel lift, but the symptoms continued. I saw the athlete when the first podiatrist was on vacation and learned that most of his running was in the hills of the San Francisco Marin County. Of course, I thought, when he puts the most stress on his achilles, he must be on the ball of his foot. So, I extended the heel lift to include the full foot, therefore the lift would work when the runner went up onto the ball of the foot. This worked wonderfully, and the patient reported 100% reduction in symptoms.

Since I have told Ben's low back pain story and the incredible success of lift therapy, I think I shall mention iliotibial band syndrome. The iliotibial band protects the outside of the hip and knee. The iliotibial band is irritated or stressed by pronation forces (which rub the iliotibial band at the greater trochanter or lateral femoral epicondyle), supination forces which stress the lateral structures of the lower extremity, and short leg syndrome which also stress the iliotibial band as it tries to straighten the leg. Short leg syndrome, aka limb length discrepancy, causes a dominance or lean in the lower extremity. This lean can cause the iliotibial band to strain as it works very hard straightening the leaning leg. Lifts to correct the short leg syndrome can be immediately

helpful in iliotibial band syndrome. Gait evaluation should be as valuable as an MRI in noting the reduction in limb dominance when using lifts on the correct leg (the short one)..

Short leg syndrome is a syndrome since so many problems develop from the problem as mentioned briefly above. As you talk to your patients, you should always get a good history of their current problem, and other problems that the past has brought their way. A runner with iliotibial band strain now, with a history of hip pain, unilateral achilles pain, and some low back pain can be a pronator, a supinator, or have a short leg. You then watch them walk, and/or run, and see if the pattern for a short leg exists. If it does, you can then do a cursory exam standing with palpation of the iliac crest heights, anterior superior iliac spines, and greater trochanters. This can set the stage for treatment that can end a patient of recurring repetitive stress injuries caused by having hips, pelvis, and spine that are not level.

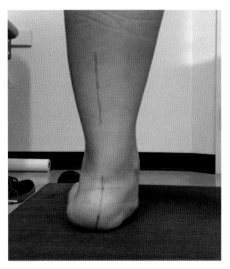

Unilateral over pronation can cause a drop in the pelvis causing a functional short leg.

Practical Biomechanics Question #502: If you measure a short right leg on the more pronated side, what are the possibilities?

Practical Biomechanics Question #503: If you measure a short right leg, but the left leg is more pronated, what are the possibilities? Answer: 709

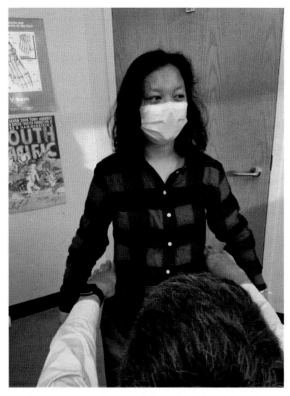

It is so important when you are evaluating for leg length that your hands are parallel, easily observable, and your head is at the level of the examination

Classic Limb Length Presentation and Treatment

The patient presented with left posterior tibial pain medial ankle for 3 months during. Rest, icing, new shoes, and 5 visits to a PT were tried to help. And, this approach was helping somewhat. The PT

sent the patient to the podiatrist for diagnosis and another PT Rx. Historical review showed other possible past pronatory issues: plantar fasciitis, big toe joint pain, shin splints, and knee pain. The patient was dealing with chronic low back pain and awaiting an MRI and possible epidural cortisone injection.

Examination showed left posterior tibial pain and gait pattern of asymmetrical more left sided pronation. Limb dominance was seen to the left side in gait. Osteopathic standing evaluation for leg length showed a short left side possibly due to flatter arch on that side. Posterior tibial tendon was sore on muscle testing and patient could not do a single heel raise due to this ankle pain medially.

The patient had at least a functional short leg with collapse of the left arch recently. This could not explain the chronic low back pain. Treatment started with ⅛ inch lift short leg, and OTC arch support (stocked in the office) left only to create a more level pelvis and help the posterior tibial tendon. This asymmetrical treatment definitely helped the low back instantly, with less effect initially on the posterior tibial tendon.

Over the next 3 months, treatment continued to rest and support the left foot arch, and lift up the left side higher. A CAM walker was used with EvenUp to really get the posterior tibial tendon under control, with the arch support and lift only on the left side. Around the house the patient wore an Aircast Airlift PTTD brace left only for about 5 months total (also dispensed from office practice).

With the early low back relief with lifting up the apparent short left side, the need for an epidural went onto the back burner. Custom orthotic devices were made with more pronatory support on the left side. The separate lift was eventually increased to ¼ inch sulcus length. The left orthotic device had a stabilizing (and lifting) external rear foot post, and the right had none.

After the Immobilization Phase was over, and the custom orthotic devices made, the patient was sent back to PT for posterior tibial strengthening (was already doing active range of motion and isometrics), and a full lower extremity program of strengthening and stretching to help with anti-pronation muscles. The PT also helped with the small amount of inflammation that still existed. Bicycling was the main form of cross training for the first six months, and then some swimming and pool aerobic exercises started with the warmer summer months.

By 7 months post injury, with the patient cross training, beginning to walk for exercise 3-4 miles, of course with lifts and more orthotic lift on the short and injured left side, the low back pain continued to be silent.

Her stage 2-3 posterior tibial tendon dysfunction was maintained for the next 10 years (until lost to followup). She remained diligent with her custom orthotics and lifts, although in that 10 year period she had two flares due to improper unsupportive shoes and no lifts.

RCSP (heel bisection) was done with and without orthotic devices. RCSP 9 everted left without orthotics and 3 everted with orthotics. RCSP 3 everted without orthotics and 0 everted with orthotics. Her pelvis remained level with orthotics and an extra ⅛ inch lift left sulcus length. Every 1 degree is about 1/16 inch. Therefore, the original 6 degree difference in RCSP was ⅜ inch difference in length of leg with left shorter since more collapsed.

Chapter 11: Weak and Tight Muscles

Stretching Principles

Practical Biomechanics Question #504: Why are we taught not to stretch through pain? Answer: 709

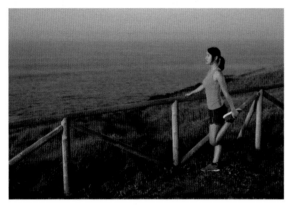

Runner stopping to Stretch left Quadriceps and Stabilizing herself by holding onto the fence

In treating the lower extremity, it is very important to emphasize stretching of the most important muscle groups: plantar arch, calf, quadriceps, hamstrings, iliotibial band, hip flexors, hip extensors, and hip adductors. Of these 8 groups, there are variations that are important like separating the stretch for the gastrocnemius and soleus while doing calf stretches. Here are the basic principles I teach. If patients learn a few at first, you can build onto these principles so that they become smart stretchers. The 14 general stretching tips are:

1. Hold each stretch 30 to 60 seconds and repeat twice. My own personal trainer uses the principle for anyone over 30, hold one second for each year you have been alive.

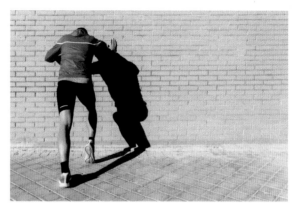

Left Calf Stretch with heel held on the ground. If the knee is straight, you are stretching the gastrocnemius muscle.

2. Alternate between sides while stretching which is easy when you are doing 2 sets of each stretch.
3. Do not bounce while stretching, you want a prolonged hold
4. Deep breathing while stretching to get oxygen into the tissue (one deep breath is equivalent to 6 seconds). A 30 second stretch is normally 5 deep breaths.
5. Stretching before activities should be done after a light warm up (do not stretch cold) especially if you exercise in the morning.
6. Stretching after a workout will gain you the most flexibility since the tissue is heated up
7. If one side of the body is tighter, do twice as many on that side to seek balance (usually one more set on the tighter side is preferred to start balancing out the tissues).

8. If you want to gain flexibility, stretch 2 to 3 times a day whether you work out or not

9. If you want to maintain flexibility, stretch once daily

10. Never stretch through pain

11. Make sure when stretching your body is stable (stretching should not be a balancing exercise also) by holding on to a wall or chair or fence.

12. Stretch the tissue in varying positions to see if you find some tightness (try to stretch and vary foot positions, amount of joint bend to start, etc).

13. If you are sore, and you can find a stretch that helps, you are on your way towards getting better

14. If stretching the sore area makes no difference, you may be stretching a tendon that is too flexible (have it measured) or the pain is more inflammatory or neurological. Tightness produced by nerve tension can be made worse with stretching and this can be diagnostic.

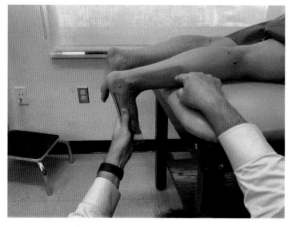

Measuring gastrocnemius flexibility

The tendon I stretch and stretch the most is the achilles tendon in my clinical practice. It is both the strongest tendon in the body, and I argue the most influential. The foot functions poorly when it is too tight, and the foot functions poorly when it is too loose. It is so important to be able to measure reliably so that you can find the pathological tight patients, and the pathological loose patients. You must understand the Force Length Curve idea of tendons, and its significance in why patients are having problems related to the achilles tendon. The basic premise of this curve is that both a tight tendon and an over stretched tendon are physiologically weak. The normal length of a tendon is called its resting length or its normal physiological length (NPL). At the NPL, the tendon is in its ideal position to develop the most power or force. We know when we measure the achilles, both the gastrocnemius and soleus have ideal lengths. In the lower extremity, the hamstrings and the quadriceps also have measurable lengths that are ideal. So, if any of these 3 tendons are off, either too stretched out or too tight, we can measure that and give treatment advice to attempt to improve the situation. See Chapter 4 in Book 2 on measuring Achilles Flexibility.

Practical Biomechanics Question #505: What are two ways to measure gastrocnemius strength? Hint: One is related to flexibility. Answer: 709

Helping with the Excessively Tight Tendons

There are 4 common techniques utilized by doctors and physical therapists when normal stretching is not helping. These are:

1. Mobilization of the Muscle Belly
2. Contract Relax Techniques
3. Various Splints
4. Prolonged Heat and Ice Constant Stretch

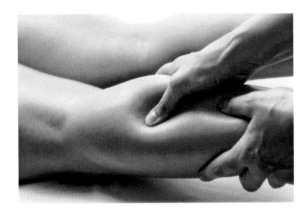

Mobilization of the Calf muscle belly for tightness

Mobilization of the muscle belly is a good way to stretch out a tight tendon. The loosening of the muscle belly is typically performed by a physical or massage therapist skilled in this treatment. It can take up to 8 sessions, and I request that the patient sees me after the 4th treatment to see if we are progressing. I have achieved good reliability in my measurement, so after one month I can tell if improvement is occuring. You get good at various measurements by standardizing how you do them, and being exact at your technique time and time again, so you can not possibly measure any other way. Many of my patients are muscle bound in some way, with muscles that seem to hypertrophy with use overnight. Even though I think of stretching and massage in the same way, deep mobilization (massage)

seems to be intense enough to really relieve that tightness in muscles. Many physical therapists will use heat or ultrasound prior to mobilization. Some use ice afterwards on the muscle belly.

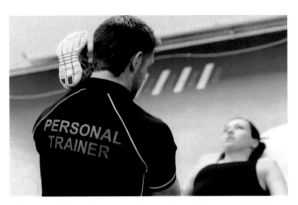

Photo of Trainer performing Contract Relax Technique on Tight Hamstrings with the patient pushing down on the shoulder and then the trainer stretching the tendon

There are various **contract relax** techniques, and some of these the patients can perform themselves. The basic principle is to contract the tendon to fatigue it (like 5 single leg heel raises), then stretch for 3 seconds (sometimes with heat), then more contractions to fatigue, then more stretching. This is never done with pain. Coaches will do it for their athletes, parents to children, or it can be self administered. Another very valued method of contrast relax means you contract the antagonist before stretching the agonist. An example is to contract the ankle extensors 10 seconds against resistance, and then stretch the achilles for 30 seconds, and repeat.

Practical Biomechanics Question #506: Explain the basic principle of Contract Relax self application. Answer: 709

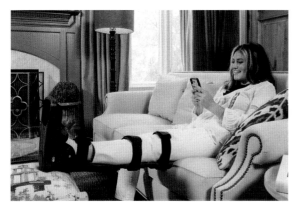

DeHeer Equinus Brace which crosses the knee for gastrocnemius stretching

We have various **splints** to wear that are now over the counter, like the myriad of plantar fascial sleeping splints that stretch the soleus and plantar fascia. The DeHeer Equinus Brace also has promise for gastrocnemius tightness. Many Practitioners have just made their own over the years, but they typically can not be adjusted once the angle is set.

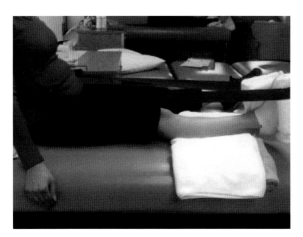

Heat Ice Prolonged Stretch Technique with the stretch maintained the entire time and a heat pack then ice pack utilized

Many years ago I started working with a Temple University design for stretching tight quadriceps post surgery. I have used the technique of **prolonged heat and then ice** for the quadriceps, hamstrings, and achilles. The principle is 2 times more heat than ice with a continuous stretch even as you change the heat pack to an ice pack. The goal is to allow the heat to stretch and lengthen the muscle, with the ice freezing the tendon golgi organs at the new length. I am not sure of the ideal amount of time, but I have always done the 2 to 1 ratio, and initially performed in my office so I can measure before and after. This needs a partner to help for the achilles for sure. I will do 10 minutes of heat and 5 minutes of ice initially, and if not helpful, advance to 20 and 10 or 30 and 15 respectively.

Strengthening Principles

Strengthening exercises are a crucial part of a lower extremity rehabilitation progress. We are either trying to just strengthen the injured area, to use strength as part of a full lower extremity program, or to prepare an athlete to return to their specific sport with specific strengthening needs. It is so important to know that muscle strength is vital support to injured bones and joints, as strengthening the surrounding muscles takes stress off of the skeletal structures. Also, when a certain muscle or tendon is injured, the surrounding similar acting muscles can help restore motion and thus speed up recovery to normal function. The Golden Rule I use is that muscle re-strengthening should begin the day before the injury (ASAP).

There are many components to a strengthening program. The podiatrist in charge of someone's rehabilitation is the best to know what muscles are injured and when the patient can begin a return to activity program. I personally like to be involved with each part of the program, at least knowing what my co-treaters are doing, and to be very specific in my Rx writing. This can become the way you learn what works and does not want. The more interchange you can have with a physical therapist, massage therapist, occupational therapist, acupuncturist, etc, the more you will help the progress go smoothly.

So, in forming a re-strengthening program, what are some of the basic components? They include:

- Type of Strengthening
- Phase of Rehabilitation
- Role of Cross Training
- Specificity of the Activity Training
- Progression of Exercises for Safety
- Overloading to Build Strength vs Overtraining Causing Reinjury
- Recovery
- Time of the Day
- Painful or Not

The various types of strengthening includes:

- Location: local, specific function, and more global
- Types: active range of motion, isometric, progressive resistance, isotonic, functional, and isokinetic

When you injure a specific spot, it is important to strengthen the local area of any muscles involved. When it is a specific muscle, you really need to strengthen all the muscles that do similar functions to help. An example of this is an injury to the posterior tibial tendon. What does the posterior tibial tendon do, and what muscles can help do the same function taking strain off the posterior tibial. The posterior tibial tendon supports the arch (anterior tibial, intrinsics, and peroneal longus), decelerates contact phase pronation (anterior tibial, flexor hallucis longus, flexor digitorum longus, gastrocnemius, soleus, lateral hamstring, sartorius, gluteus medius and minimus), and assists ankle plantar flexion (previous muscles and peroneus brevis). So, with a posterior tibial tendon injury you are not only strengthening the posterior tibial but many other muscles to help take the strain off that particular muscle/tendon. I definitely feel the injured muscles should be individually strengthened, but the others can be strengthened more globally in bigger motions (usually done with functional activities). You can see how important it is for muscle strengthening routines that the prescriber must know muscle function, some quite complex, and a slew of good safe exercises. Since there are good, unsafe in some way, exercises, you have to be aware of some of the possible problems with a certain exercise.

Practical Biomechanics Question #507: What is most difficult to do for a patient right after they are injured: isotonic or isometric exercises? Answer: 709

The **type of strengthening** should match up with the **phase of rehabilitation** that the patient is in. These phases are Immobilization, Re-Strengthening, and Return to Activity. In the Immobilization Phase, active range of motion and isometric exercises are typically well tolerated. In the Re-Strengthening Phase, progressive resistance and isotonic exercises should be tolerated. In the Return to Activity Phase, strengthening continues with more functional strengthening with less isolation and more isokinetic or advanced isotonic. The exercises should not only match the phase of rehabilitation, they should not get in the way of the rehabilitation. This means the exercises should gradually and progressively get the patient stronger while not causing a breakdown with increased demands.

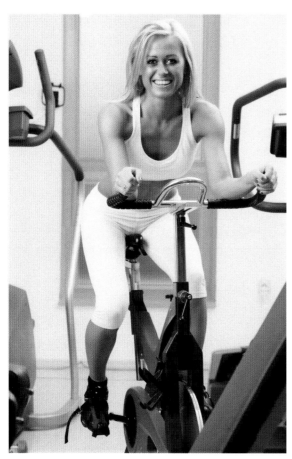

Cycling, in its many forms, is one of the most utilized Cross Training techniques

Cross Training, the use of other exercises to maintain strength and cardiac condition, are the bookends in this progress. Bookends support the right and left sides of the books, or mark the beginning and end of a progress. Cross Training keeps the body strong both at the beginning and end of the progress. For runners, cross training when they can not run may be cycling, swimming and elliptical. For dancers, it could be walking and pilates. When you are developing a cross training plan, you have to decide on the Impact vs Non-impact, Cardio or no Cardio, motion of the injured area or no motion to the involved area.

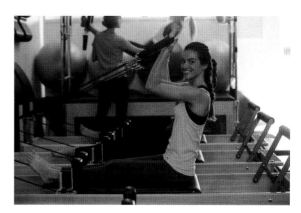

Pilates Cross Training for Injured Dancer

The **specificity** of the program of re-strengthening concerns the goals the patient is going towards. Are they runners, dancers, walkers, cyclists, or just concerned with getting back to daily life? Is it tennis, singles or doubles? Is it basketball? Or is it a 500 mile trek through Spain? This is where specificity is needed with the injured athlete or patient. Designing programs to help a basketball player slowly return to the courts, a dancer to the stage, or a hiker to the trails in the High Sierras, is an incredible task. Some podiatrists are Phase I doctors, but I enjoy the full program. Starting to finish is a fun journey with my patients.

The **progression of exercises** in a rehabilitation process means that we work the muscle through more and more strenuous exercises as safely as possible. Due to our normal body rhythms, the strengthening may go good one day and be less effective the next day. The easiest strengthening exercises can be done daily, and the more arduous ones only every other day. The patient will have to sense when they need to progress every other day due to the difficulty of the exercises attempted. Simple active range of motion and isometric exercises can and should be done daily, even several times a day, and can/should be started as soon as possible in the event of injury. Both of these exercises can also be done without and with gravity to add some extra difficulty. The invisible hand of gravity working against an exercise may feel at times as a resistance band blocking motion. The patient is then progressed into progressive resistance exercises using sports cords or resistance bands. These should be done during the start of the Re-Strengthening Phase, and continued into the Return to Activity Phase. There are normally 6 color bands noting increased tension. The athlete progresses through (will be explained later) from 2 sets of 10 at level 1 to 2 sets of 25 at level 6.

Practical Biomechanics Question #508: What is a benchmark for strengthening and how is it established for a patient with resistance bands? Answer: 709

The concept of **Overload** should not be mixed up with the concept of **Overtraining**. Overload builds up and Overtraining breaks down. Overload is a way to stress the tendon so each week you get stronger and stronger. This is the goal I set for my patients and they can easily visualize their progression with the levels of resistance bands. This is done by increasing the sets and repetitions done of an exercise gradually. Overload can not hurt, but icing after exercises in case of too much load is recommended. Overloading a tendon is done with the watchful eye of a physical therapist or personal trainer. Overloading can be done gradually, albeit slowly, as a defined home program. Overtraining is very wrong, but walks in the disguise of improvement. Overtraining does not have enough recovery time between events. Overtraining fatigues the muscles too much and re-injury can occur. Overtraining will show a steady or sudden decline in performance. Overtraining may also accompany higher resting pulse rates, restless sleep, or increase in muscle soreness, and actual injury.

Recovery is as essential for athletic performance as the time training for a certain event. Most high level athletic events, like basketball, are only done 3 times a week for good reason. The reason is that recovery time allows for all the micro-injuries to heal, and not an actual injury to occur. Sports like football have found 7 days between maximal athletic performance gives the athlete time to heal (thus the erroneous nature of Thursday night football). Yet, recovery is used for every injury and every individual no matter the age. We need time to recover. Whereas maximum performance may be once a week for football, and three times a week for basketball, every 5th day for a baseball pitcher, physical therapy twice weekly for an injured athlete, and ankle resistance bands every other night, it is important to find the level of an activity that one can do relatively safely and at their best. This delicately maintains some overloading to strengthen, without overtraining to re-injure.

Practical Biomechanics Question #509: As an injury gets better, rehabilitation procedures must allow some pain to enter the equation. What does it mean when an athlete is allowed to participate as long as the pain is back to normal in 2 days? 709

Time of the day makes a big difference in strengthening exercises. In treating lower extremity injuries, you really do not want to fatigue the injured area and then have to use it a lot. I prefer to have my lower extremity exercises, where I am trying to gradually make the patient stronger, be done in the evening. That way when they fatigue their muscles, especially the injured ones, they have all night long to rest. This can be hard for my patients that prefer to exercise in the morning, but they adapt.

Practical Biomechanics Question #510A: Why is lower extremity evening strengthening preferred? Answer: 709

The last general rule for strengthening is **not to strengthen through pain**. It is so important to never break this rule while stretching. And typically, this is the general rule for strengthening. But, tendons like the posterior tibial with its adjacent posterior tibial nerve, seem to hurt a lot while strengthening. And swollen areas, at times, can only get stronger by exercising through pain. So, the treating doctor or physical therapist has to analyze how the painful exercise may affect the patient's feelings that day and the next day. Sometimes the pain will linger for 2 or 3 days and therefore not recommended at that time. Strengthening can be a balancing act.

There are some of my general strengthening rules:
1. Begin to strengthen the day before an injury happens or the day before the patient sees you for the first time. This emphasizes the immediacy of beginning strengthening. ASAP seems not soon enough.
2. Even though injuries have a definite period of Re-Strengthening, strengthening should begin immediately and continue well after the injury is finished.
3. Strengthen not only the injured area but also above and below the injured area. One of the best examples is patellofemoral syndrome where strengthening needs to be at the knee, but equally important at the hip and foot.
4. You should consider a removable boot, ankle foot orthotic device, foot orthotic device, brace, and taping all part of the Immobilization Phase in an injury until the body gets strong

enough to not need these devices. Of course, for many reasons, some assistive aid like orthotic devices may become permanent but that should not minimize the need to stay strong. For example, patients in stage II PTTD who are trying to avoid surgery may always be in orthotic devices or some other braces, while they daily keep all the anti-pronation muscles strong.

Practical Biomechanics Question #510B: What are the 8-9 top muscles to strenghten to slow down the foot pronation? A: 710

5. Since podiatrists deal with over pronation syndrome constantly, strengthening should consist of foot intrinsics, posterior tibial tendon, anterior tibial tendon, peroneus longus tendon, gastrocnemius and soleus muscles, pes anserinus tendon group, and external hip rotators like gluteus minimus, gluteus medius, iliopsoas, and piriformis.
6. Since podiatrists deal with over supination syndrome constantly, strengthening should consist of both peroneal tendons, stretching an overly tight achilles tendon, and strengthening of the hip adductors, medial hamstrings while making sure the lateral hamstrings have normal flexibility, and strengthening of the internal hip rotators.

It is important to talk here about the 2 hallmarks of the Re-Strengthening Phase: Progressive Resistance Exercises and

Functional Exercises. Progressive resistance is something I am explaining daily to my patients and a great way to begin to build up an injured muscle/tendon. Functional exercises are something that physical therapists reign supreme and begin to prepare the patient to get back to their normal activities. These are the two types of exercises that generally prepare our athletes to return to activity.

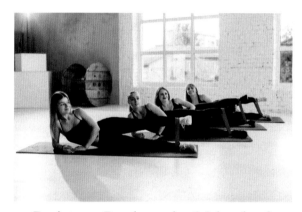

Resistance Bands can be 6-8 levels of resistance and can be used for all lower extremity muscles

I love progressive resistive exercises for my athletes. I want to start these as soon as possible for most activities. Prepare the patients on their first visit by starting to activate their muscles with active range of motion both without and with gravity. You normally just begin to tone the injured area this time, and your overall rehabilitative program will grow and grow. Active range of motion is at its easiest allowing gravity to assist or at least have no influence. Consider the ankle muscles with their six directions of muscles: plantarflexion, dorsiflexion, inversion and eversion to start, with dorsiflexion with inversion or dorsiflexion with eversion to round out the 6 directions.

Practical Biomechanical Question #511: With the 6 main ankle motions above, what muscle is strengthened with each? A: 710

Imagine the downward pull of gravity working on these muscles. For the first week, each evening, have the patient do these 6 ankle directions, by not fighting gravity. Typically, active range of motion is 20-30 exercises or repetitions in each direction for one set. From a normal sitting position, plantarflexion, plantarflexion and inversion, and plantarflexion and eversion will be easy. The 3 directions which involve a dorsiflexion force will have to be done with the patient lying on their side to avoid the influence of gravity. The next 3 motions then are dorsiflexion, dorsiflexion and inversion, and dorsiflexion and eversion. If all goes well, and the patient can progress, these 6 directions must fight somewhat against gravity. Now, from a normal sitting position, the 3 dorsiflexion motions easily fight gravity, with the plantar flexors lying on your stomach, and both inverters (dorsiflexion and inversion, and plantarflexion and inversion) and everters (dorsiflexion and inversion, and plantarflexion and eversion) on alternating sides. You want the individual motion to pull up towards the room ceiling when lying on their back and pulling upwards towards the knee for the dorsiflexion motion. It is so important to understand that injuries, or pain itself, causes an immediate shutdown in muscle activity.

When, or if, active range of motion exercises are easy, you can begin isometric. This is typically in the third week ideally, but at least the next step in the process. Isometric means toning the muscle while it remains in its same length. So, you contract the muscle as you push against an immovable object. With the 6 ankle directions, this can be challenging, but not difficult. Patients with good flexibility use their hands, while others have to use opposite feet, the bottom of a couch, or just a stiff sports cord applying good resistance to prevent motion. You could also do this with and without gravity, but I primarily have the patient find the best position to apply the resistance in each of the 6 directions. Isometrics are typically 2 sets of 10 repetitions. You contract the muscle for 6 seconds against the immovable object, relax for 4 sec, and repeat 10 times. Rest then 5 minutes and repeat. Since you have to find all 6 positions, it normally takes about 5 minutes to go through the first set anyway. As with active range of motion, there should be no pain, and can be done twice daily. After 2 weeks of active range of motion, and 2 weeks of isometrics, most patients are ready of progressive resistive exercises. Some of this will depend on who you are having to show these exercises and when their upcoming appointments are.

Theraband ® is one of the original companies that makes these rubber bands that can be used to provide gradually more resistance to movement. They are numbered level 1 through 6, usually each one with a different color, with the

Practical Biomechanics Question #512: Explain how to do AROM dorsiflexion exercises without and with gravity. A: 710

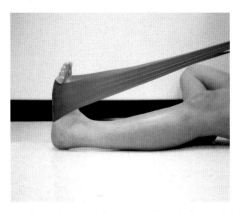

Level 3 Resistance Band for ankle plantarflexion which can be done in 2 positions (knee straight and knee bent)

patient instructed to progress through the levels easiest to hardest. If you are putting a patient on a general 6 directional ankle program, they are encouraged to start with 2 sets of 10 for each direction. Normally, they are tasked to find out what motions are the hardest and what motions are the easiest to do. I will soon talk about the normal progression through the levels, and some of the muscles can easily progress daily through the early levels to find where they should be. It is normal that one patient is at one level with the posterior tibial tendon, another level with the achilles tendon, and another level with the peroneus tertius and extensor digitorum longus. Many patients just strengthen around the weakest one (by staying with that resistance band for all exercises), and other patients are doing different levels for different tendons which can take record keeping and a certain complexity.

When you do 2 sets of an exercise, it is important to do the first set easier (activating the muscle and warming it up), and the second set with a little more tension

in the band. This general rule is not done with weights normally, but the resistance bands provide an easy way of adding a slight amount of more tension. This is why as you go up in repetitions, you typically go up first with the first set only (the warm up set) to get your body used to the increased load. You start with level one 2 sets of 10, then one set of 15 one set of 10, then 2 sets of 15, then one set of 20 one set of 15, then 2 sets of 20, then one set of 25 one set of 20, and finally 2 sets of 25. Each of these levels should be done at least 3 days and typically only after band 2 should you change to every other day to do these exercises. Bands or levels 1 and 2 typically can be done daily, but levels 3 and higher should have a rest day between.

So, to summarize the progression of resistance bands:

1. Level 1 two sets of 10
2. Level 1 one set 15 one set of 10
3. Level 1 two sets of 15
4. Level 1 one set 20 one set of 15
5. Level 1 two sets of 20
6. Level 1 one set 25 one set 20
7. Level 1 two sets 25
8. Level 2 two sets of 10
9. Level 2 one set of 15 one set of 10
10. Level 2 two sets of 15
11. Level 2 one set 20 one set 15
12. Level 2 two sets 20
13. Level 2 one set 25 one set 20
14. Level 2 two sets 25

This progression continues through levels 3 through 6, and then a bike inner tube can be utilized (although some of the companies have come out with 8 levels. If I have a patient with posterior tibial tendon Stage 1 or 2, and I want to prevent progression, they need to build their way to 2 sets of 25 at Level 6 (as one common podiatry example). Or the chronic ankle sprain patient with weak peroneals that needs to build up to 2 sets of 25 Level 6 for both the peroneus longus and peroneus brevis tendons.

Practical Biomechanics Question #513: After level 4 two sets of 20 repetitions, what would the next progression be of resistance band? Answer: 710

Practical Biomechanics Question #514: If you are doing 2 sets of a resistance band, how much time should be between each set to rest? Answer: 710

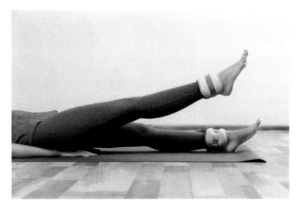

Isotonic Strengthening means that there is Same Weight (here set weight for hip and knee isotonic strengthening exercises)

The last part of re-strengthening that I get involved in for my rehabilitation programs are isotonic. Isotonic and functional exercises occur mainly in the world of physical therapists and personal trainers. Isotonic means the same weight is applied. You set the weight to be moved and then you move through some range of motion or exercise. The motion has to be smooth, not jerky. Your typical single leg

press for patellofemoral problems is a great example. Another common example are hamstring curls with set weight. The development of programs for patients using the Single Max Rep is crucial for great muscle development and the understanding of progress made. You can really begin to see that in rehabilitating a patient you want 3 crucial things to happen: pain stays at 0-2, function returns to pre-injury levels, and the strength of the area involved and the whole limb is improved. For most injuries at the foot and ankle, there are no direct isotonic exercises to do. Even for foot injuries, you normally want to make the knee and hip stronger, so isotonic exercises may be part of the overall plan. If isotonic exercises are being prescribed to an area recently injured, or in pain, I prefer a physical therapist in charge. If the isotonic exercises are being prescribed to another area for overall muscle strength, personal trainers are preferred.

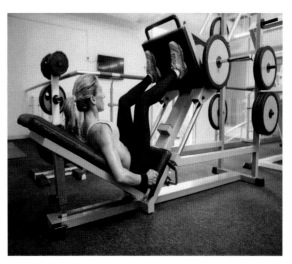

Isotonic Quadriceps Strengthening (here two sided isotonic can easily become one sided by releasing one side)

Practical Biomechanics Question #515: Doing a single leg press for patellofemoral joint pain patients, should your foot be straight or turned out slightly? Ans: 710

I will end my discussion on strengthening with functional exercises. The discussion so far in this chapter on strengthening has been on isolating muscles to get stronger, finding out where they can be strengthened safely, and progressing them through a program. Functional exercises can be safely started in the Re-Strengthening Phase of Rehabilitation and begin to prepare the athlete or injured patient for the next phase where they return to full activity. Functional exercise is also called functional training and works groups of muscles together. You exercise the muscles and neural pathways to begin to re-group and become a baseball player again or conquer normal daily activities, after sometimes months and months of immobilization, and sometimes after surgery. The therapist or trainer must analyze the movement patterns needed in the next phase, break them down into simpler forms of movement, and then progress the patient. You can imagine the skill level not only needed by a trainer rehabilitating a basketball player, which can be relatively simple, to someone trying to conquer 20 steps in a two story house (which can be a monumental task). When I think functional exercises, I think core. The core muscles must stabilize the lower extremity and assist their finite movements. When I think about functional exercises, I think movement patterns that neurologically need to be reset.

Functional exercise brought into rehabilitation whole new ways of thinking about muscles and the nerves that innervate them. I love the concepts of movement patterns, muscle activation, and core which all became extensions of this concept. What are movement patterns? What is muscle activation? What really is core and its importance in podiatry?

It is important for an athlete to begin to break down the stresses of their sport, and design a gradual return to full activity protocol. Consider the early stages of a basketball player's rehabilitation when they maybe can only shoot free throws since their lower extremity can be basically immobile other than a slight knee bend. But, they have to be able to bend their knee and ankle and load the front of their foot. What does each skill require? Do they have the range of motion, flexibility, and strength to begin?

When we rehabilitate a patient, we not only have to be concerned with forward motion (no limping as we watch them walk), but also with the other basic movements patterns of lateral motion, weight transfer from left to right, up and down motion, and the coordination of the upper and lower body. Testing our strength with functional exercises should include how well we can perform these basic movement patterns. If we fail today, exercise programs are designed to move us towards success, or have a legitimate reason for our failure. When failures occur, why must be asked, and then Plan B developed, new imaging, consult with the physician, etc.

When we rehabilitate a patient, we have to be aware of the fundamental movements patterns needed in life. The common patterns are needed for day to day activities include:

- Walking
- Bending
- Reaching
- Squatting
- Running
- Kicking
- Shifting Sideways
- Moving Around People and Objects

It is important to test the patient and see if there are any defects in abilities. If so, set a new benchmark to achieve and work towards it. As you send your patients to rehabilitation, especially those following surgery or severe injuries, ask the PT what the patient's limitations are in the basic movement patterns. These limitations have to be assessed in the early part of rehabilitation.

Practical Biomechanics Question #516: Following an achilles rupture and successful surgery or cast immobilization, what must be assumed in terms of the overall achilles tendon strength the first day of rehab? 710

I look at the concept of muscle activation as waking up a lazy muscle. There are experts in muscle activation to call upon for help. I get my first clue when I am testing muscles and the patient is slow to respond to my command to fire the muscle into my hand. I have personally found that the common active range of motion exercises are great at this task of muscle activation. But, it can get complicated, where expert

care is needed. Pain can be a real downer when it comes to strength gains. If moving a muscle produces pain, the patient will typically avoid the movement and the muscle atrophies. So, part of muscle activation comes from allowing muscles to move through pain when appropriate, so they will not decondition and shut off. After an inversion ankle sprain for example, the tendon may be fine, but because of all the swelling, the peroneal tendons hurt to move. These muscles then stop working, and the patient is more at risk for another ankle sprain. Here muscle deactivation can be the primary cause of a worse second ankle sprain. This is but one example.

Practical Biomechanics Question #517: What is one reason due to muscle strength due we place ankle sprains in an ankle brace for a while? Answer: 710

Another reason for muscle deactivation can be neurological, both measurable and subtle. The nerves that protect an area in pain unconsciously stop those muscles from working, since their activity causes pain. The nerves can also be damaged from other causes. The damage can be measurable or not, and the injured nerve can cause a delay in how the muscle it innervates works. Why is this important? Most injuries have acute or overuse causes. In rehabilitating these injuries, you want the involved muscles to work well. If the common muscle is deactivated, due to a secondary neurological deficit, it is not going to help you much. In the foot, these neurological deficits are commonly from the L3/L4, L4/L5, or

L5/S1 nerve roots. Treating foot problems can commonly need help from the back.

Practical Biomechanics Question #518: In evaluating foot function, a patient was found to have poor FHL tone. What spinal disc could be involved? Answer: 710

What is core? Core is the midsection. Core is vital to the foot. Core work strengthens and stretches vital muscles to the foot. You have to look at the foot as part of the whole body, and the proximal leg and core as a way to lift you off your foot. The stronger and more powerful the core, the overall less stress in movement on the foot. The core basically lifts you off the ground. If you treat feet, make sure that a physical therapist works the core at the same time as the feet.

So, as a patient strengths from an injury to help them move through the rehabilitation phases, it is so important that the following occurs:

- The muscles involved are isolated
- The functional exercises are used
- That the core in engaged
- That problems with muscle deactivation are corrected
- And remember, weakness and tightness are always linked

This quest may lead to other issues to be explored and treated. We, of course, have to recognize that some of our patients are motivated, and will make changes, and others will not. I believe in setting the bar high for each patient and seeing where you go. Patients may surprise you in both ways, either super compliant or totally not connected to the program.

Chapter 12: Poor Shock Absorption and Various Instabilities

Poor Shock Absorption

As I watch a patient walk, I define them into five categories which have served me well in my investigation into why they might have symptoms. From there, I try to correlate those findings to their symptoms and then treatment options. The five categories are: overpronators, over supinators, limb length discrepancy, weak and tight muscles, and finally poor shock absorption. What can cause you to be a poor shock absorber? The most common gait, and then biomechanical findings, that cause poor shock absorption are:

- Excessive contact phase supination
- Rigid foot type with reduced subtalar joint motion
- Patient functioning at maximal subtalar joint pronation (so no pronation available for shock absorption)
- Pes Cavus Foot Type with Increased Heel Strike

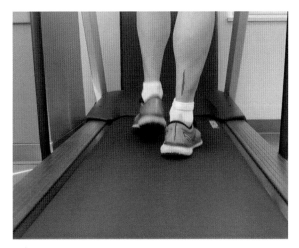

In a Patient with Poor Shock Absorption, you may see no heel motion

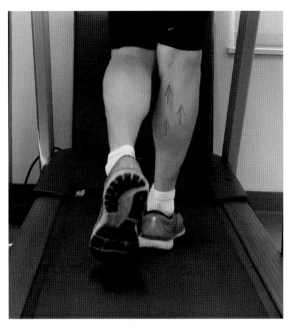

In a Patient with Poor Shock Absorption, you may see a shock wave going up the calf

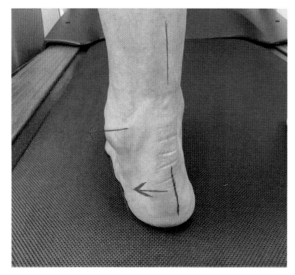

In a Poor Shock Absorber, you may see Heel Contact Supination with lateral Drift of the lower leg

Practical Biomechanics Question #519: Poor Shock Absorption can be part of a patient's intrinsic biomechanics, or just part of the mechanics of their activity. Discuss prolonged downhill running as a cause of poor shock absorption. Answer: 710

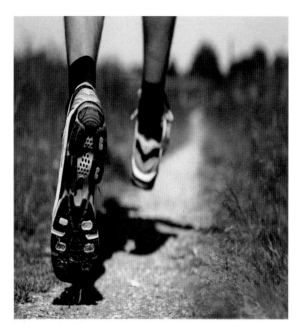

The need for shock absorption gets getting the faster you run

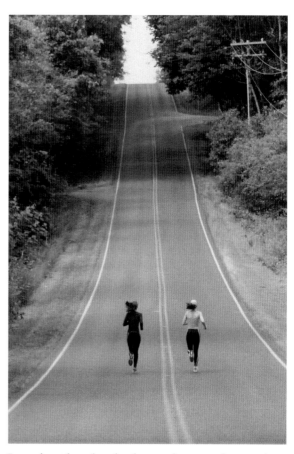

Imagine the shock absorption needs running down this hill

Even though you can use the softness of shoes to get some shock absorption, this type of treatment will tend to backfire with the excessive supinators, maximally pronated patients and pes cavus feet. Softness begets instability especially when there is inherent instability already present. Every podiatrist who treats patients in this arena has a list of stability shoes and neutral cushioned shoes to give their patients. This is the time to use those shoes that sort of cross over into both categories, a sort of stable cushioned shoe. As of this writing in 2023, my favorite in this category is the Brooks Ghost.

Poor Shock Absorption leads to jarring problems with stress fractures and joint arthralgias. If the poor shock absorption is from contact phase lateral instability, supination problems can be common also. If the poor shock absorption is from functioning in a maximal pronated state, pronatory symptoms can be part of the presentation. You have to go back to Chapter 9 (in this Book 3) to review both pronation and supination syndromes.

Practical Biomechanics Question #520: What blood test should always be taken when a patient presents with an overuse related stress fracture related to poor shock absorption? Answer: 710

Practical Biomechanics Question #521: How does an osteopenic bone density make you more prone for a stress fracture with high impact loads? Answer: 711

I typically tend to improve my patient's shock absorption in two ways: reverse the poor biomechanics with custom orthotic devices or use the Hannaford memory foam full length orthotic device. These treatments will be explored next in Book 4 Chapter 13 on orthotic devices and their components. Yet, what other common treatments are there for a patient with a jarring gait and femoral or tibial stress fractures? These treatments are all part of a biomechanical approach to a patient. These treatments include:
- Softer Shoe
- Various Methods of Decreasing Contact Stress
- Softer Insert
- Total Contact Supportive Insert
- Environmental Factors

- Training Factors

Practical Biomechanics Question #522: I learned years ago that a hard piece of plastic can be an incredible source of shock absorption? Explain how a plastic orthotic device can help absorb shock in a runner.

Softer shoes can be very helpful in managing shock absorption issues. For the patients who fit that category, the shoe softness may have to be in the heel only, the forefoot only, or the whole foot. The heel is important when you are trying to reduce impact shock in a heel striker. The forefoot is important when you are trying to reduce impact shock in a forefoot striker or someone always on the balls of their feet. The full foot cushion is more important in walking and standing activities where there may be equal amounts of time on the heel and forefoot. Softness has to be balanced with stability as there is typically a loss in stability by degrees as you add softness. Running shoe stores are very helpful pointing patients towards the most appropriate shoes, but have to be helped by expert advice. Simply writing where the stability and cushion need to be on a RX pad can be helpful.

Practical Biomechanics Question #523: In the orthotic/shoe world, if you have a very unstable shoe, the orthotic will help gain some stability. What type of orthotic device would you need in a very stable hard shoes like the Brooks Beast in a patient with chronic tibial stress fractures/reactions? 711

Decreasing contact stress consists of many methods to lower the ground reactive force that has to be absorbed by the body. It is discussed a lot in running, but also plays a role in the rehabilitation of many activities and shock related injuries. After a knee or hip replacement, these concepts form a valuable framework for activities moving forward. Even though a part of the other factors just mentioned (softer shoes, softer inserts, total contact inserts, environmental factors and training factors), decreasing contact stress can encompass everything one does in life. After an injury, it may be soft shoes and taking one step at a time. Or the runner with repeated leg stress fractures, may be told only to run down hills gingerly, never, or only at the start of a run. Or the young football player needing a hip replacement at 30 being told not to run, but to become a world class cyclist. So, decreasing contact stress, becomes the patient's mantra for life, and expresses itself in many forms.

Practical Biomechanics Question #524A: Why can it make a big difference for a runner to run the downhill part of a course first instead of at the end (in terms of the development of stress fractures)? A:711

Softer inserts typically have neopreme (like Spenco® Products), or poron®, or plastazote® (memory foams). With the softness you can get some instability over 1⁄8 inch, and some durability issues with memory foam products. When patients have pain on the bottom of the foot, these soft inserts should be against the foot if possible. But, if you are treating knee or hip arthralgias with these shock absorbing materials, they can be put under an orthotic for example.

Total contact supportive inserts work to distribute weight evenly throughout the foot during the contact and midstance phases of gait. Most orthotic laboratories now know and do make orthotic devices that support the foot well making good total foot contact with the subtalar joint in neutral position. However some feet seem to have problems with this in the manufacturing process. Typically these are the pes cavus feet or the feet with high degrees (over 6-7 degrees) of forefoot varus. Full support of these feet tend to cause other issues, so hybrid orthotic devices with some less support are made. My common solution for this problem, if I can recognize it before the first pair of orthotic devices are made, is to begin orthotic therapy with Hannaford devices. These total contact orthotics are made of various densities of plastazote® material, and hybrids with other forms of material can be made and experimented with. When a shock wave enters the bottom of the foot, unimpeded it will travel up the leg towards the knee. The straighter the knee, the more that stress enters the knee, hip and low back areas. We can imagine that shock wave of ground reactive force being vertical. Anything between the ground (where it is going to enter the foot), and the foot that runs perpendicular to that force can help dissipate the force. Here shoes and orthotic devices, even ones with very thick rigid plastic, because they run perpendicular to the force of ground reaction can magically help reduce that force.

If you can indulge me with a little physics, Pressure = Force applied/Area in which the force is applied. The force is ground reaction force. The area is increased by increasing the surface that the force must act on (an entire foot and orthosis and shoe). The pressure exerted by ground reaction is therefore diminished by common modalities.

The one common exception that I commonly deal with are the application of heel posts or lifts with patients who are heel contact strikers. This can be anything designed to focus forces at the heel, even heel lifts. When ground reaction force hits the heel, and there is a dominant heel piece (even the heel of a dress boot), the force can increase up the leg over barefoot, and not be dissipated. Patient feedback is crucial, and subjectively, the patient should not feel either that the heel is clunky at contact, or there is more jarring to the leg at contact.

Environmental factors are many depending on what sport or activity is being played or enjoyed. Patients that already have poor shock absorption due to their intrinsic biomechanics have to be serious about controlling these vital other factors. How the environment affects shock absorption is either in adding hardness at impact, or poor positioning with increased supination motion or pronatory position. If you think of a banked trail with one foot being held pronated and the other supinated across the subtalar joint, you can imagine the supinated foot losing the needed pronation of shock absorption and the pronated foot maxed out so that there is no pronation left to help absorb stress.

Broken down shoes, a definite part of a runner's daily environment, can hold feet too pronated or too supinated, or no longer provide good shock absorption. When you live in San Francisco, like I do, or another city with many hills, this vital part of the environment can lead to too much stress, particularly running downhills. Researchers have found that strong muscles protect bones. This is fairly straightforward. Athletes in training can go through times when their muscles are tired and less protective to their bones and joints. Also, during a long run, it has always been advisable to have the downhill segment at the earlier part of the run when the muscles are more protective. It is also common knowledge that the cement in sidewalks is harder, and more jarring, than the asphalt in the street. That is not completely true since cold asphalt, say at 5 am, can be as hard as cement, but warm asphalt on a hot afternoon can be 7 times softer than cement. Any time you are the doctor for a local sports team you have to consider the environment of the athletes. I remember working with a gymnastics club and getting them to research and buy better mats for the children, and advising on training workouts for my cross country teams, and getting rid of hard astroturf for a baseball team. These recommendations come from treating the various injuries year after year and trying to decide the root cause(s). Remember, the root cause is normally 3 causes coming together (Rule of 3).

Practical Biomechanics Question #524B: What are several possible ways that a runner can decrease the shock stress to the legs if vulnerable for stress fractures? 711

Training factors have been looked at before, but I want to highlight the common problems I see in practice. One of the biggest issues that end up jarring our joints is poor recovery times. Typically, hard workouts need 36 hours to recover, and older individuals like me need 48 hours to recover. Without that recovery time, our muscles have less and less ability to protect our bones and joints. Triathletes have pushed the envelope of training with the 3 sport routines: running (mainly lower extremity impact), cycling (mainly lower extremity non impact) and swimming (mainly upper body strengthening and lower body stretching). By rotating these 3 sports, basically stressing various aspects of our bodies with each sport, they can train and recover very well. Runners can vary stresses well with longer slower runs, shorter and faster runs, hill runs, etc. Runners can also vary their shoes. Since this is the section on shock absorption, staying away from useless long downhills on training runs is crucial, and varying the terrain as much as possible is very important. Trying to get quality over quantity seems the best in your training advice. I personally think if athletes varied their shoes from traditional, to Hoka® style ones, to minimalist (racing), the varying stresses would cut down on the overall injury rates.

Two of my best shock absorption stories concern the Hannaford orthotic device which I hope you are familiar with or have a comparable device (it will be discussed in the next chapter in Book 4). The Hannaford orthotic device was invented by running guru Dr. David Hannaford when he practiced in Eugene, Oregon. Eugene is renowned as the running capital of the world. After Dr. Hannaford introduced the orthotic around 1986-87 at an American Academy of Podiatric Sports Medicine meeting, I had a patient that seemed to fit the bill. She was a nurse from Oakland, California, and had attempted three times to run a marathon only to break a bone at each time about 17 miles into her training. The three separate breaks included the femur twice and the pubis bone in the pelvis. When I watched her run, I noted what a pounder she was, someone with poor shock absorption and no foot motion noted at the heel. She fit my criteria of being poor at shock absorption which would be the cause of her stress fractures. I told her about the Hannaford orthotic device and she was willing to try. 10 years later when I last was in contact she had successfully run 7 full marathons of 26.2 miles.

My second example was a referral from a fellow physician. This patient had broken his femur running 3 times, each with 6 to 9 months of rehabilitation. Again my gait evaluation revealed someone poor at shock absorption. After fitting David for his Hannaford designed orthotic devices, I did not see him for 3 years. For the next 3 years he had run the most mileage ever totally injury free, until another femoral stress fracture occurred. He called somewhat complaining that #1 he probably had another stress fracture, and #2 wasn't the orthotic devices designed to prevent that. When I got to see him again, his Hannaford orthotics were like pancakes. I explained that they probably need to be modified once a year, and remade every two years, to keep their protective function.

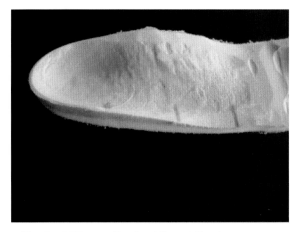

Typical Hannaford without the top cover designed with 2 one half inch layers of plastazote ® vacuum pressed

I would be remiss if I did not talk about bone strength. As I have explained earlier, injuries are produced by 3-5 factors coming together (Rule of 3). The goal is to have the practitioner not just blame one thing as the cause of an injury, but look for other causes. It is easy then to play Sherlock Holmes when a patient gets an injury. If you discover the causes(s), you will speed up the rehabilitation and prevent recurrences. The patient can avoid reinjury. So, when we talk about an injured patient with poor shock absorption, what could be going through your head?

- Did they deserve it somehow by overtraining?
- How did they cause so much stress to their body to cause an injury?
- Can we change their shoes to have a positive effect?
- Can we change their inserts to have a positive effect?
- Can we change their form or pace in any way?
- Can we change the terrain they move on, or anything else about their training?
- What is the health of their bones if they broke it? Or the health of their joints, if they are stressing them out?

Common Serious Lower Extremity Instabilities

What instabilities do we want to explore? This is my 6th category that I define patients under. They can usually be defined by another category already listed, but the presence of these observed instabilities, seen in your typical gait evaluation, and the potential damaging effects on a patient are worth highlighting and trying to get to the bottom of. Remember, as a podiatrist, you may be the only one picking these problems up, sometimes years before symptoms, and you can do incredible good work in helping them. These instabilities commonly seen in gait that deserve this extra attention include:

- Excessive Lateral instability
- Genu Recurvatum
- Excessive Internal Femoral Rotation
- Pelvic Instability
- Varus Thrust at Knee
- Unilateral Hip Hike

Part of the reason that they fall into their own category of gait findings is that some of these findings could require surgery down the road, or at least produce significant disabilities. Therefore, we are not just talking about helping a marathoner run 26 miles, but potentially delaying or preventing a major surgery, or major disabilities. Most of these have been explored in the previous chapter on gait evaluation, but deserve another mention. What are the potential risks for each? These include:

- Excessive Lateral Instability leading to Ankle Reconstruction
- Genu Recurvatum leading to Achilles Lengthening or Full Knee Replacement
- Excessive Internal Femoral Rotation leading to knee, hip and back problems
- Pelvic Instability leading to Hip Replacements or Spinal Surgery
- Varus Thrust at the Knee leading to at least Partial Knee Replacement Medially
- Unilateral Hip Hike leading to Hip Replacement Surgery or Chronic Low Back Pain

Are the surgeries inevitable? Sometimes they are, sometimes they can be prevented, and sometimes they can be delayed. I love delaying big potential surgeries as long as the patient is out of pain and fully functional, since hip and knee replacements have a life of 15 years and if you do the math on a 45 year old, how many surgeries will they have in their lifetime? If I can delay the first to 55 or 65, they will have much less trauma to their bodies, and much less chance of complications.

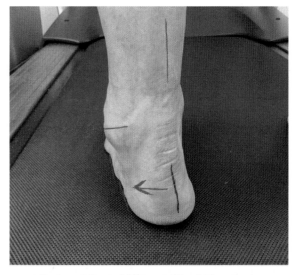

Lateral Instability at Heel Contact

Lateral Instability is a very unstable gait. The foot strikes the ground, and instead of rolling into its normal pronation for shock absorption and ground adaptability, the foot supinates. It may be something that happens barefoot, only with shoes only, only with certain activities, and or only with orthotic devices on. This is why I always watch patients walk, and run if they run, and in various shoes. Chapter 9 highlighted the types of complaints you will hear from the patient who excessively supinates (aka lateral instability). It may happen after an ankle sprain that weakens either the lateral ankle ligaments or the protective peroneal tendons. It may be in a patient that has a high degree of tibial varum, but typically pronates, until their shoes break down when worn too long. So, for patients with lateral instability noted in gait, the checklist I go through to discover the cause(s):

- Everted Forefoot Deformity (like plantar flexed first ray or forefoot valgus)
- Tailor's bunion with unstable fifth ray

- Excessive Pronation producing unstable cuboid or lateral column (typically with another cause of lateral instability)
- Lateral Ankle Ligament Instability
- Peroneal Weakness
- Laterally worn down shoes from tibial varum or excessive external angle of gait
- Favoring of the Opposite Leg
- Excessive External or Internal Angle of Gait
- Unstable or Laterally Broken Down Shoes
- Over corrected Orthotic Devices

If we can identify the problem, fix it, we can prevent the devastating problems associated with lateral instability, and potential surgery down the line.

Practical Biomechanics Question #525: What are 7 common causes of lateral instability in patients that can cause problems? Answer: 711

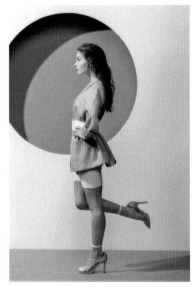

Standing with Genu Recurvatum (mild here)

Genu Recurvatum (sway back knee, locked knee) is a very destructive problem at the knee where the tibia locks back on the femur. It is caused by either a primary knee problem, ligamentous laxity, or tight gastrocnemius. It is primarily seen on the side view of the knee, which is a part of gait evaluation that I do not do routinely. In gait, you can see that the knee looks straighter than normal, especially at push off. At times, when the patient is standing in front of you, as you look for possible genu valgum, etc, you will see them hyper-extending the knee joint. And, when you check for ankle joint dorsiflexion, you may observe the knee hyperextend as the body tries to relax the gastrocnemius and give a few more degrees of ankle bend. Children with genu recurvatum from a congenitally tight gastrocnemius should have a few months of stretching, followed by a gastrocnemius release if the conservative care is unsuccessful. If the genu recurvatum, also called sway back knees, is related to ligamentous laxity, then both hamstring strengthening and prolotherapy to the knee capsule should be entertained. If the genu recurvatum is primarily a knee deformity in the sagittal plane, improved hamstring strength is primarily encouraged if there is no pain. They must get into the habit of standing with a "soft" knee, which is a knee slightly bent. They gain stability by locking the knee back, but making this a long term habit is very bad for the knee overall.

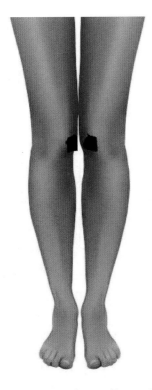

Excessive Internal Patella positioning (Squinting Patellae) with the black marks indicating kneecap bisections

Excessive Internal Femoral Rotation is a destructive transverse plane force causing terrible foot pronation, awkward knee malalignment, and all the symptoms of these 2 problems. Chapter 9 highlighted the problems related to abnormal foot pronation, and the knee malalignment causes terrible positioning problems. With the knee too internal, the medial knee is unstable and torqued, and the lateral knee joint too compressed. The famous Q angle (quadriceps angle) is too high, and symptoms will occur. The patient may stand normally, but when they walk or run may have too much internal femoral rotation. When standing alone shows the problem, it is called "squinting patella" with the kneecaps looking at each other. The treatment can be mainly from the foot,

mainly from the hip, or both. Inversion placed into a foot orthotic device is important to generate enough rotational force or supination moments to decrease the internal femoral moments. Attacking this problem at the hip with a strong external hip rotator strengthening program is vital.

Practical Biomechanics Question #526: What does a simple varus wedge at the foot due to the knee alignment in a patient with excessive internal femoral rotation? A: 711

Pelvic (postural) Instability is noted as you watch someone walk and the lateral or side to side sway of the trunk is accentuated. When a patient is starting to have issues, this sway may simply appear as limb dominance. Limb dominance is one of the signs of having a short leg problem and the trunk will stay over the long or short leg for most if not all of the time in gait. I have discussed this in the preceding chapter on leg length, and the chapter on gait evaluation. However, as you watch someone walk with beginning postural instabilities, the dominant leg side will vary, sometimes the drift is to the right and sometimes to the left. The patient may unconsciously drift to one side of the hallway meaning as they walk away from you they will lean to the right (for example), and as they walk towards you they will lean to the left. The two classic usual neurological forms of postural instability that I see are: Trendelenberg from weak Hip Abductors (could have some neurological form), and the sway from a painful arthritic hip. The difference between these two is simple: Trendelenberg forces the trunk to fall away from the support leg, and with an arthritic hip the weight goes over the painful hip in the support phase. This is of course different if the patient is limping in an acute problem, just lending to the good side. Postural instability is an exaggerated sway of the trunk either away from the supporting leg (Trendelenberg) or towards the supporting hip (arthritic or painful hip). A good referral is then made as you most definitely have been the first to make these diagnoses based on your routine gait evaluation of patients.

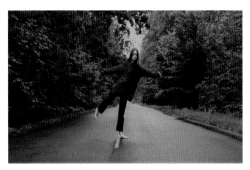

Painful Hip will have the trunk longer over the support leg longer

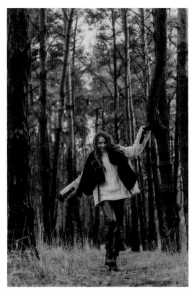

Trendelenberg falls to the non-supportive side

Varus Thrust Knee is a very damaging force. The medial knee compartment can be damaged with this problem. As the foot strikes the ground, the knee jerks into increased varus with the proximal tibia compressing the medial femoral condyle.

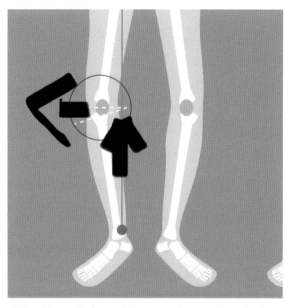

The Knee Joint will move Lateral, and the Medial Joint Line will be compressed in Varus Thrust

This breakdown can lead to greater and greater genu varum deformity and eventually a knee replacement. I wish the knee always just responded to my corrections at the foot. But, the knee joint can be influenced by hip motion, foot motion, or its own independent axis of motion. I do not think that we know if it is the motion itself or speed of motion that does the most damage. I try my best to change the forces across the knee joint when treating these patients with various types for orthotic devices: valgus wedge anti-supination ones when appropriate, varus wedge anti-pronation ones when appropriate (counter intuitive but successful over 50%), and Hannaford shock absorbing inserts just to decrease the shock absorbing role at the foot.

Practical Biomechanics Question #527: Medial Knee Compartment problems are typically extension issues, and Lateral Knee Compartment problems are typically flexion issues. Explain why keeping the knee slightly flexed can help medial knee joint line pain. Answer: 711

As you watch the patient walk, after noticing the varus thrust, notice if there is any abnormal knee motion that working on hip muscles may help. The biggest example of this is the presence of internal femoral rotation at the same time as the varus thrust (which may be helped by external hip rotator strengthening and lateral hamstring strengthening to externally rotate and flex the knee), or some limb dominance over that knee that lifts to correct a short leg may help. Perhaps, just strengthening or stretching appropriate weak or tight muscles/tendons may be very helpful at the knee or hip if found. A good gait evaluation finding of varus thrust at the knee, which can occur many years before symptoms, and many years before the patient would seek any sort of treatment, can start the patient on conservative treatments which may help incredibly. You are making a great observation that can help the patient in years to come if you can start simple treatments.

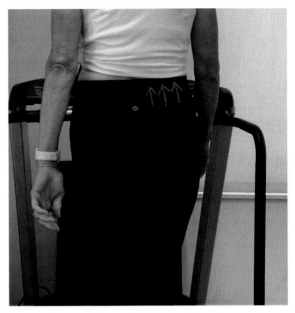

Hip Hike is seen following Foot Strike with a Jerk to the hip upwards at the time of foot loading

Unilateral Hip Hike is primarily seen as the patient walks away from you in your gait evaluation. The transverse or sagittal plane hip motion following foot strike should be symmetrical and smooth. Therefore, a unilateral upward jerk at the hip at foot strike is very dramatic. From a podiatrist standpoint, it means something is happening up at the hip area. I wonder if sometimes all I am seeing is the good hip moving and the bad hip stuck and not moving. Patients with this have been diagnosed with longer legs on the side of the hip hike. They have also had arthritic hips and jammed up sacroiliac joints. When you make the observation, and whether the patients have symptoms or not, consider an orthopedic or osteopath referral. I have several great osteopaths in my area to make these priceless referrals. A change in the body's ability to compensate for a long leg, due to sudden weakness from illness or another problem, or a shift in weight due to another problem (even unilateral arch collapse or knee replacement for example), or just the slow core weakness that sets in over time, and all of sudden there is a problem seen on gait evaluation.

Practical Biomechanics Question #528: Gait evaluation can be a key to discovering abnormalities years before symptoms. What problems may be associated with the gait finding of Hip Hike? Answer: 711

Answers to Self Corrected Chapter Questions

Chapter 7

#324: What are the 3 Phases of Rehabilitation? What Phase typically uses casts? What Phase typically begins a Walk/Run Program? Immobilization, Re-Strengthening and Return to Activity. Immobilization. Return to Activity

#325: Why would heel lifts help patients with anterior ankle impingement? Help clear anterior ankle in stance

#326: Why would a weak achilles tendon cause anterior ankle impingement pain? Ankle does not plantar flex late in stance jamming anterior ankle

#327: Explain why heel lifts work in anterior ankle impingement syndrome? Help clear anterior ankle as tibia moves forward on the talus

#328: Tallmenshoes.com can add 3 inches to men's height. When would you use this for anterior ankle impingement syndrome? All the time when patient wants to wear dress flats

#329: What crowds the front of the ankle more–traditional running shoes or zero drop shoes like Altras? Zero Drop

#330: Explain why stretching the foot extensors can ease stress in the front of the ankle joint. Relaxing the ankle extensors means less dorsiflexion the ankle, so less anterior ankle crowding

#331: Mobilization techniques are Graded 1-5. What Grade would you do when there is a lot of pain in the ankle, and what grade would you do with no pain in the ankle? Grades 1-2 with alot of pain, Grade 5 if no pain.

#332: Would plie or releve in ballet irritate the anterior ankle in anterior ankle impingement syndrome? Plie

#333: Which of the following is not for correcting lateral instability. There can be more than one answer.
1. Deep Heel Cups
2. Denton Modification
3. Valgus Wedging
4. Kirby Skives (medial or lateral)
5. Rearfoot post motion (x)
6. Forefoot Varus Support (x)

#334: When you compare the heel to ball relationship during a prolonged downward dog to standing achilles stretch with the heel dropped off a platform, what in terms of body weight stress or force moments are different between these two exercises? Standing with heel off platform (negative stretching) puts the entire column of body weight over the ankle.

#335: When taping the achilles tendon, is the goal to limit the ankle bend completely? No

#336: When a patient has anterior ankle impingement, what are the classic exercises to do? Heel Raises

#337: When a ballet dancer began to get anterior ankle impingement symptoms, what positions (plie or releve) were immediately removed from practice? Plie

#338: When you think that a patient functions too inverted, especially with contact phase supination, what are 2 muscles to check for weakness? Peroneus Longus and Peroneus Brevis

#339: What is the typical resistance band progression after 2 sets of 20 for both the peroneus longus and brevis tendons? 1 set of 25 followed by 1 set of 20. Alternate between the 2 tendons.

#340: Would a low or high ankle sprain benefit the most from an Aircast Stirrup Brace and why? Low Sprain needs inversion protection

#341: Why do patients with narrow heels need higher cam walkers? Narrow heels swim around in the lower cam walkers, and you need the velcro to go high up the leg to stabilize

#342: What is the chief difference between typical crutches and Canadian crutches? Canadian crutches have pressure on the hand, wrist and forearm

#343: When applying a valgus wedge to a shoe, you have to watch a patient walk with the shoes on. What motion are you trying to prevent? Over supination called lateral instability

#344: Name 6 common orthotic prescription components that can be used in lateral instability patients. High heel cup, lateral phalange, no post motion, Denton modification, lateral Kirby skives, forefoot valgus correction

#345: In an attempt to begin strengthening of the peroneal tendons, the patient started doing 2 sets of 10 repetitions Level 1 resistance bands in what 2 ankle positions? Ankle plantar flexed and ankle neutral (right angle foot to leg)

#346: Single Leg Balancing is a common exercise taught for ankle, knee, hip and low back rehabilitation. How long are these positions typically held? Build up to 2 minutes

#347: When addressing ankle instability, why would some patients only wear braces when playing sports? Braces restrict muscle function, so should only be worn when needed to prevent sprains

#348: There are so many boots that can be worn year long if needed to help lateral ankle instability. What can you add to a boot to help lateral ankle problems? Foot inserts like orthotic devices, taping, and ankle braces

#349: You could just focus your whole career on Achilles injuries; it is such an important structure. What are the 2 muscles

that make up the achilles tendon?
Gastrocnemius and Soleus

#350: We can gain so much information on the state of the achilles tendon by measuring its flexibility and strength. What does it mean when ankle joint dorsiflexion is 30 degrees with the knee extended in prone non weight bearing measurement? That the gastrocnemius is overly flexible and therefore very weak

#351: Explain why in the case of an undiagnosed micro tear in the achilles tendon, continuing to keep the pain level 5-7 is not an ideal protocol? The fragile healing of the microtear most likely will keep re-injuring and never completely heal

#352: There is debate on whether single leg balancing or a heel raise is the most important exercise every patient should be doing. How much do you have to bend the knee to begin placing the stress on the soleus and off the gastrocnemius muscles? The knee bend only has to be 15-20 degrees to elicit the soleus.

#353: When you think mechanics, you should think in terms of how your mechanical changes affect the lower extremity in both positive and negative ways. Explain why a heel lift placed in a shoe puts increased stress on the plantar fascia, but this is minimized by a heeled shoe. As a shoe insert, the heel lift ends right where the plantar fascia begins, therefore we lose some plantar foot support there. A heel as an intrinsic shoe component

allows the entire plantar foot to be in contact with the shoe.

#354:The TC Angle between the tibia and calcaneus is also called the Achilles Angle. O degrees is where the tendon and heel line up perfectly. It is not uncommon to run with an Achilles Angle of +20 degrees (very pronated). Treatment therefore should be directed towards more varus positioning of the heel. What are 3 common methods of improving this varus positioning? Kirby skives, varus posting intrinsic and extrinsic, and Inverted Technique.

#355: Review the definition of the 3 Grades of Calf Strain. Grade1 is slightly inflamed or with microtearing. Grade 2 is a partial tear. Grade 3 is a complete tear of one of the calf muscles.

#356: Injured muscles tighten up and this can be a cause of re-injury or just prolonged rehabilitation. Sports Medicine is built on a Foundation of early mobilization, including early strengthening and stretching of the tissues. What would be 4 key points to emphasize to the athlete at your first encounter to begin safe stretching? No pain while stretching, no bouncing while stretching, deep breath while you stretch, do not stretch unless you are warmed up

#357: Many deep calf strains are caused by soleal weakness with over flexibility. Match that up with over knee flexion in a runner with tight hamstrings. Why do tight hamstrings cause us to use our soleus muscle much more than the stronger gastrocnemius? As we bend our knees with tight hamstrings, the gastrocnemius is taken off stretch, and the soleus is required to do more of the work of the achilles tendon.

#358: If tight achilles/calf muscles are a cause of injury, why do we use heel lifts in their treatment which also can tighten the tissues? Heel lifts can relax the calf muscle in the short term, helping the situation. And, of course, hopefully the achilles stretching works well to get the tendon stretched out.

#359: What is Occam's Law about treatment for shin splints? Related to overuse, using ice to calm down, will improve when the muscle strength catches up to the activity.

#360: Which of the following is false regarding muscle testing.
1. Always test muscle strength early in the day x
2. Always compare both the right and left sides
3. Examine a muscle both where the examiner has the advantage and the patient has the advantage
4. Test muscle strength even when there is severe pain x

#361: Match the potential overload with the various shin splints listed.
- Lateral Shin Splint
- Medial Shin Splint
- Anterior Shin Splint
- Posterior Shin Splint
1. Excessive supination due to pes cavus (Lateral)
2. Excessive strain due to a weak achilles (Posterior)
3. Excessive pronation in pes planus (Medial)
4. Excessive downhill running (Anterior)

#362: What motion of the ankle tests for the peroneus longus tendon? What motion of the ankle tests for the posterior tibial tendon? What motion of the ankle tests soleus over the gastrocnemius tendons? PL with eversion and ankle neutral. PT with inversion and ankle plantarflexed. Soleus with ankle plantarflexion and knee bent.

#363: We stretch to warm up tissue, attempt to reduce overly chronically tight tissue, and relax a sore area. Why would a muscle get tight when it is being overworked, like the anterior muscle group with too much downhill running? If a muscle is starting to strain, it begins to tighten as it heals microtearing and collects inflammatory fluid.

#364: On a steep downhill, a hiker will start hurting at their weakest link. What is being strained in the act of going downhill when there's too little fat pad under the metatarsal heads? Skeletal structure

#365: One of the best recommendations with patients with shin splints is to slow down or rest and cross train for a short time. If you think the medial shin splints are related to FDL overuse, what OTC device is helpful? Budin Splints

#366: Any case of medial, lateral, or anterior shin splints that is not improving in one month time should have what test

(besides x-rays) to look at bone health?
Vitamin D Blood Test

#367: What are the 4 common overuse tibial stress fracture locations, and which one is commonly related to over pronation? Posterior tibia (related to over pronation), distal medial tibia, proximal medial tibial, anterior tibia.

#368: Why would subtalar joint motion be implicated in tibial stress fractures? Why would an inverted heel in RCSP possibly cause a tibial stress fracture? Inverted calcaneus and talus crowds the medial talus leading to stress risers in the distal medial tibia and even the proximal medial tibia.

#369: All stress fractures have to be evaluated for torque and shock. Gait evaluation walking and/or running can typically help you decide what to do, but when the patient hurts, may have to be postponed. What are 3 biomechanical observations made just by having the patient stand in front of you that could indicate over pronation when running? Why should they bring in old worn down shoes for you to look at? Everted heel, prominence of the medial arch, tibial varum, internal patellar positioning. Worn down shoes may show how their biomechanics break down shoes like excessive medial wear in pronation patients.

#370: Why is some contact phase pronation good for shock absorption? Need pronation of the foot to act like a car shock absorber.

#371: Why in sports do heel cushions work less effectively than with standing activities? In sports, the athlete may be completely on the metatarsals and off the heels.

#372: Are isotonic exercises more powerful than progressive resistive exercises? Yes

#373: Why would a tight achilles tendon cause the development of an anterior tibial stress fracture? With a tight achilles, the ankle extensors have to work much harder getting body weight forward. They pull hard, and if the tibia is weak, can crack the tibia by this strong muscle contraction.

#374: Why does habitually running against traffic cause pronatory problems on the right leg of runners? When running against traffic, the right foot is pronated and the left foot is supinated due to the bank of the road.

#375: If we are designing an orthotic device to prevent excessive supination, why is a forefoot valgus deformity better to support than a forefoot varus deformity? Supporting a forefoot valgus is like placing a large platform under the lateral side of the foot for supination support.

#376: My first case was of a patient with a fibular stress fracture on his right side. Was he habitually running with or against traffic? Against

#377: Tape has also been known as "flexible casting" and can be very powerful at helping patients. I love to tape my athletes, and there is usually a way that can help any injury you face. Where does leukotape start medially when stabilizing the lateral ankle? Just under the medial malleolus

#378: Explain how an ankle brace can take pressure off an injured area by limiting muscle contractions, compared to the principle of limiting motion in one area can create motion or stress in another area. Both of these hold true so you want to brace only when you have to.

 #379: As you narrow your base of gait, the tibia gets more varus positioned to the ground, increasing the lateral stress on the ankle and leg. As you widen your base of gait, the tibia gets into a more valgus position to the ground, increasing the medial stresses on the ankle and lower leg. This is the same pattern with over supination and over pronation of the subtalar joint. Explain then how narrowing the base of gait is like excessive supination of the subtalar joint in its effect on lateral ankle stability. With both narrowing our base and over supination tendencies, we stress the lateral ankle making us use the lateral ankle muscles more (which can fatigue and strain).

#380: The pain from PFD can be excruciating where McConnell taping is too uncomfortable. As the symptoms calm down, McConnell taping can be vital in the rehabilitative process. Explain why the patella naturally will subluxate laterally. The naturally stronger vastus lateralis develops more power over the weaker

vastus medialis and pulls the patella laterally.

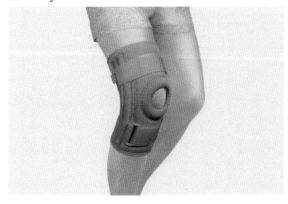

#381: What is the main purpose of the two velcro straps in the knee brace above? The velcro straps are mainly to prevent the knee brace from slipping down while exercising.

#382: What are 7 common general rules for stretching any muscle/tendon complex?
1. Hold each stretch 30 to 60 seconds and repeat twice. My own personal trainer uses the principle for anyone over 30, hold one second for each year you have been alive.
2. Alternate between sides while stretching which is easy when you are doing 2 sets of each stretch.
3. Do not bounce while stretching, you want a prolonged hold
4. Deep breathing while stretching to get oxygen into the tissue (one deep breath is equivalent to 6 seconds). A 30 second stretch is normally 5 deep breaths.
5. Stretching before activities should be done after a light warm up (do not stretch cold) especially if you exercise in the morning.
6. Stretching after a workout will gain you the most flexibility since the tissue is heated up

7. If one side of the body is tighter, do twice as many on that side to seek balance (usually one more set on the tighter side is preferred to start balancing out the tissues).

#383: Is it tight medial or lateral hamstrings that increase internal knee rotation? Medial

#384: What are common causes of not being able to stretch out tight muscles? Congenital tightness and Neurological tightness

#385: Which of the following hip muscles does not help patello-femoral tracking issues?

1. Adductor Longus x
2. Piriformis
3. Gluteus Minimus
4. Iliopsoas
5. Sartorius

#386: The motion of the knee joint is both simple and complex. Since the motion of the knee joint is influenced by 3 areas, how it responds to a certain treatment may not be predictable. What are the 3 primary areas that affect knee motion? Hip motion, foot motion, and its own axis

#387: Braces cause a positive biofeedback loop. Braces cause proprioceptive awareness of the knee while wearing. Explain how this proprioceptive awareness can help in the injury rehabilitation. With heightened awareness of the knee, the patient tends to better avoid activities that are irritative.

#388: How does one normally avoid the negative effect of braces which can cause us to lose muscle while wearing them? By only wearing them when they help avoid knee pain (which shuts down muscles even faster)

#389: Name four simple but effective knee strengthening exercises that Podiatrists can start the patient on while waiting to begin Physical Therapy treatment? Active Knee Range of Motion, Isometric (called Quad Sets), Progressive Resistance Bands, and some functional exercises like short arc Squats

#390: As we place a varus correction at the foot in an attempt to open up the lateral knee joint, what muscles must we strengthen to protect against overdoing it? Peroneals, medial hamstrings, adductors

#391: Working with Hannaford orthotic devices for the last 35 years has taught me most of their uses. They are the king of Shock Absorption. Why were they originally designed for runners? Due to being full length, the runner would never land on the front edge (like plastic) which can be irritative and injurious

#392: Medial or varus wedging of the foot can have a great effect on pes anserinus problems. When would you make the wedge longer than just a heel wedge? This depends on the part of the foot the patient spend their time on. For example, a runner up on the ball of the foot needs the wedge to go under the ball of the foot.

#393: Explain why the control of pronation can differ in orthotic design between various runners based on their strike patterns. Runners are typically easy to stabilize as their pronation happens at foot strike. Your correction must be at the heel in a heel striker, the midfoot in a full foot striker, and the ball of the foot in a forefoot striker

#394: What 3 muscle groups make up the pes anserinus? Adductors, Hip Flexors, Hamstrings

#395: What is the classic mechanical reason why a weaker than normal hamstring muscle can cause knee pain? There is a subtle muscle balance between quadriceps and hamstrings. If the hamstrings are weaker than normal, the quadriceps overly extend (or straighten) the knee. Typically anterior knee symptoms occur from this.

#396: When would you prescribe a double leg press versus a single leg press? This is totally based on pain so the two legs can share the weight.

#397: I repeat over and over to the students I teach that their treatment of knee, hip and low back problems can be very crucial. What are the 2 main reasons foot over pronation can produce lower hamstring pain? Over pronation can cause increased knee flexion tightening the hamstrings. Tight hamstrings can straighten the natural lordotic curve in the back producing pain. Also, over pronation can lead to dorsiflexed jamming of the first metatarsal blocking the

normal propulsion that needs first metatarsal plantar flexion.

#398: What does subtalar joint supination do at the knee joint closed kinetic chain? Subtalar joint supination causes knee extension (while the knee should be flexing) and a varus compression of the medial compartment.

#399: In Chapter 1 Book 1 the concept of Rule of 3 was introduced. It basically means that 3 different potential causes of an injury can create the "Perfect Storm" and the injury occurs. Explain 3 or 4 reasons why a patient in an overuse situation can develop lower hamstring pain. The hamstrings are weak intrinsically, the hamstrings are tight (therefore, relatively weak), and the training holds the knee too flexed for too long.

#400: With the main function of the iliotibial band to stabilize the lateral side of both the knee and hip, it is easy to see how injuries occur. In a patient with limb dominance to the left, what side would tend to develop IT Band symptoms? This is sort of a trick question as both sides can strain as they attempt to right the ship or "Leaning Tower of Pisa". But, if you were to answer one side, the left (the side of the dominance) is taking the most strain from overload.

#401: Why do women tend to get IT band symptoms more at the hip than men? Wider pelvis than men.

#402: We have long known in medicine that fractures can be produced by excessive pounding and by rotation torque placed on the bone. Explain several other factors related to bone injuries that are common problems. Vitamin D Deficiency, Osteopenia or Osteoporosis.

#403: Why is switching from running down hills at the end of runs to the beginning of runs helpful for femoral and most stress fractures? Muscles protect bones, but less when they are fatigued.

#404: When standing with a quarter inch short right leg, what leg would you typically lean on when there is no pain? The most compressive forces are on the long left leg.

#405: Why does increasing pronation at heel contact help in shock absorption in the leg? Pronation is the natural shock absorber at foot contact

#406: What motion of the hip is decelerated, or reduced, when applying a varus wedge under the heel in the shoe? Internal rotation of the hip

#407: Why is hip joint pain sometimes helped with varus wedges, and sometimes with valgus wedges? Varus and valgus wedges work to remove several degrees of motion of the hip joint in the transverse plane mainly. The loss of this motion, if it jams the hip joint in its end range of motion, can cause less hip pain. Also, if the wedges tend to center the hip, there is less strain from opposing muscles that try to move the hip.

#408: Name muscles that help prevent excessive foot pronation motions that could jam the hip joint into a maximally internal rotated position. Iliopsoas, sartorius, gluteus medius and minimus, piriformis

#409: Upper Hamstring problems can be sciatic nerve problems in disguise. Explain the comment test for sciatic nerve symptoms. Straight Leg Test

#410: What is the position of the knee at the time of an acute injury to the lower hamstring versus the upper hamstring? The lower hamstring is typically hurt when the knee extends from a slightly bent position. The upper hamstring is hurt when the knee extends from a really bent position.

#411: Explain the concept of Triple Crush on the nervous system in a piriformis patient that overly pronates, hyper-extends her knees while standing at work, and stretches her achilles by standing off the end of her stairs. Triple Crush implies that there are 3 common irritants to the sciatic nerve. The sciatic nerve is over stretched with the ankle maximally dorsiflexed. The sciatica nerve is stretched when the knee is straight. The tarsal tunnel, the posterior tibial nerve part of the sciatic nerve, is stretched when the foot pronates.

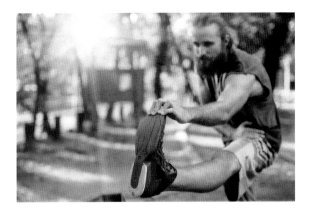

#412: Explain how this exercise (shown above) may put stress on the sciatic nerve. The sciatic nerve is stressed with ankle dorsiflexion, knee extension, and hip flexion.

#413: Patients that you are treating biomechanically will have back pain/SI joint pain. What 4 mechanical changes were discussed in the preceding section may help? The treatment for back/SI joint pain commonly treated by Podiatrist: limb length discrepancy, contact phase supination, functional hallux limitus treatment, tight hamstring treatment, and excessive pronation treatment

#414: What are the 5 main gait signs that someone may have a short leg causing lower back pain? Head tilt, shoulder drop, dominance to one side, uneven belt line, asymmetrical arm swing or lower extremity function

#415: Theorize the pros and cons of using a heel lift as your only treatment for leg length discrepancy. Using heel lifts is technically the easiest treatment for shoe fit, however when the patient functions on the metatarsals, the heel lift gives no LLD treatment.

#416: If the mantra for treating Short Leg Syndrome is "Start Low and Go Slow" why did Maurice in the preceding story have ⅞ inch lifts placed on all his shoes immediately? The impatience of youth

#417: When we measure (by many methods) that one foot pronates twice as much as the other side, which foot is acting as the short leg? The more pronated one since the plantigrade lowering of the arch will lower the pelvis on that side.

#418: How does excessive pronation cause an apropulsive gait in some patients? How does that apropulsive gait potentially cause low back pain? Apropulsive gait means no push off. If your foot can not push off, the low back get be jerked at the end of midstance leading to low back pain.

#418: What does it mean to have both medial and lateral instability? How could that affect your treatment for low back pain? Medial and lateral instability occurs in patients that have both pronation and also supination tendencies. Since both pronation and supination can cause low back pain, correcting both at the same time is important. This can take compromise in your orthotic Rx.

#419: What parts of a standard custom made functional foot orthotic device could cause low back pain and why? Any aspect of a custom orthotic device that goes under the metatarsals, and possibly toes, can block the forward motion of the foot temporarily and jerk the low back. Also, you want to support the foot and not cause contact phase supination which can irritate the low back. If a standard orthosis causes low back pain, look for signs of over supination. Thirdly, the heel post can jar the back and may need to be removed. Ask patients with low back pain if they like wearing heels or flats more.

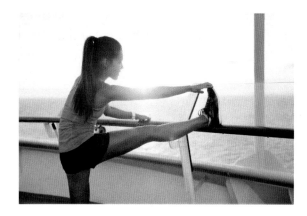

#420: What are the two main types of Hamstring Stretches, and which one is demonstrated in the photo above? There are upper and lower hamstring stretches with the lower hamstring stretch demonstrated above.

Chapter 8

#421: With Dr Root and colleagues, they were trying to establish a reference point for biomechanics and subsequent treatment in their classifications of normalcy and deformity. "Normal" was really "Ideal" in that there would be no deformities causing pathology. How did they attempt to measure a forefoot to rearfoot deformity? Placing the subtalar joint in neutral position, maximally pronating the midtarsal joint, and then measuring the relationship between the heel bisection and the forefoot plane across the metatarsals.

#422: If the deformity is a high degree of Tibial Varum, what would the normal compensation be at the foot? Subtalar joint pronation with calcaneal eversion to attempt to get the heel in a vertical position.

#423: If the deformity is a first metatarsal too high (metatarsus primus elevatus), what would the compensation be at the rear foot? Heel eversion to bring weight onto the first metatarsal head.

#424: When a neutral suspension cast is taken (in subtalar neutral and midtarsal joints maximally pronated), what are the 3 types of forefoot alignments found? Forefoot perpendicular to heel bisection, Forefoot inverted to heel bisection, and Forefoot everted to heel bisection.

#425: Dr Root taught balancing frontal plane deformities by taking a good impression cast was key to many foot problems. What could a tight achilles or weak posterior tibial tendon cause to complicate the stability Dr Root was seeking? Dr Root taught that his functional foot orthotic devices would not work when there were weak or tight muscles. These problems would have to be remedied.

#426: What are the 3 rockers of the foot allowing smooth forward motion during the stance phase of gait? In the contact phase it occurs through the first rocker, where the rounded shape of the heel allows the reception of body weight to be transferred forward. In the middle stance phase the second rocker is produced with the ankle joint allowing the tibia to move forward to transfer the load to the forefoot. Dr Dananberg cites the importance of the take-off phase, because it is when the foot, in a closed kinetic chain, transfers the body weight to the other foot, that the swing phase begins. This lever fulcrum allows the entire weight of the body to be transferred thanks to the capacity of the metatarsophalangeal joints (the third rocker), especially from the first metatarsophalangeal joint.

#427: If functional hallux limitus can be the precursor to degenerative changes in the big toe joint, what advice should you give all your patients who present with functional hallux limitus? I would advise them that for daily activities, and especially high impact, that they should always have inserts or padding that reduces the functional hallux limitus.

#428: What are the 5 common compensations that individuals will take when they have difficulty bending their big toe joint at the start of the propulsive phase of gait? These 5 common compensations include:
1) Alteration of the takeoff of the heel
2) Toes raise in phase takeoff
3) Reverse Step
4) Adduction or Abduction in phase Take-off
5) Knee and Low Back compensation of the body

#429: What is the number one treatment for functional Hallux limitus? Kinetic Wedge ®

#430: The movement from our heel at foot strike to the end of push off should be smooth. Any block in that motion will give problems somewhere in the body. When in gait does the low back get the most stressed according to the Sagittal Facilitation Theory? At heel lift (beginning of Take-Off Phase)

#431: Manter's classic work laid the foundation 80 years ago of the midtarsal joint having many axes. How many did he believe existed and what were their names? The long axis and the oblique axis

#432: The Van Langelaan study showed that the axes of foot joints were of what type? Helical

#433: Christopher Nester concluded that the midtarsal joint only has one axis that moves in all three body planes. By removing the concept of a longitudinal axis of the midtarsal joint, how does a forefoot supinatus or pronatus develop? Single axis would have representation across all three body planes, with the anterior-posterior part of the axis giving frontal plane motion and joint dysfunctions.

#434: Whereas the exact measurements are a bit confusing here, needless to say, the one axis of the midtarsal joint theory makes sense. What are the 4 main joints below the knee which help in forward motion? Ankle joint, subtalar joint, midtarsal joint, and big toe joint.

#435: Foot joints have axes that allow motion in all three cardinal planes, and thus called triplanar. Axes that are more vertical allow a greater amount of what type of motion? Transverse plane

#436: What are the 3 types of stress that can cause injury to our patients? Compression, traction, shearing

#437: McPoil and Hunt really changed how some people felt we should be treating patients. Whereas orthotic devices described by Root and Dananberg work well with this concept, the emphasis of Tissue Stress is on what treatment modalities? Reducing the load stress on a tissue by any means.

#438: The plastic region to the rupture point can be applied to tendons, bones, and ligaments. What structure when damaged can have the most long lasting and devastating problems? Ligaments

#439: Chapter 2 in Book 1 discusses the thought process of when to image, how to keep pain between 0-2, etc. Many injuries, like ankle tendonitis syndrome, have superficial pain when the problem is really deep. Explain the concept of when a superficial complaint is not getting better why you should think "deep". Problems deep under the skin are the hardest to diagnose. They can present with pain above them, or closer to the skin. If the treatment of a condition is not improving, consider looking deeper for another source of the patient's pain.

#440: Chapter 1 of Book 1 (and then later in Chapter 2) discusses the Rule of 3 which helps in our model of how an injury occurs and how we can treat that injury. Discuss a possible Rule of 3 for big toe joint pain (many examples exist). The Rule of 3 means that there are typically 3 causes of pain. In the case of big toe joint pain, the causes can be medial overload by excessive pronation, joint malalignment from a stage 3 bunion or dorsiflexed jammed first metatarsal, and mild to moderate arthritic changes within the joint. The rule of 3 also implies that one of the treatments may be the most important for that individual patient: toe separator or CorrectToes® for joint alignment, orthotic devices for pronation control, joint cleanout for the arthritic changes.

#441: The tissue stress concept typically uses many modalities to help reduce stress. What would 5 modalities commonly used to reduce stress in an injured posterior tibial tendon? Taping, PTTD brace, varus bias orthotics and shoes, and changing the activities participated in.

#442: What 5 treatment modalities can be utilized to reduce stress in an achilles injury? Biking instead of walking, taping, CAM walkers, heel lifts, lowering seat on bike

#443: What 5 treatment modalities commonly used to reduce stress on a big toe joint injury? Biking instead of running, spica, offloading orthotic devices, skip shoe laces over the big toe joint, CAM walker for weight bearing activities for a certain amount of time.

#444: Force applied perpendicular to a joint axis produces what percentage of compression forces, and what percentage of rotation forces? Force vectors acting on a joint axis with one direction perpendicular to its moment arm will resolve to 0% force compression and 100% strength rotation.

#445: What are Newton's 3 Laws?
1) Newton's First Law, sometimes referred to as **the law of inertia, describes the influence of a balance of forces upon the subsequent movement of an object**.
2) Newton's second law states that the net force applied to an object is equal to the mass of the object times the acceleration of the object.
3) Newton's third law states that for every action (force) in nature there is an equal and opposite reaction.

#446: Explain the basis of a Free Body Diagram on the ankle joint axis.
A free body diagram is defined as follows: A free body diagram is a graphic, dematerialised, symbolic representation of the body (structure, element or segment of an element) in which all connecting "pieces" have been removed. The only rule for drawing free-body diagrams is to depict all the forces that exist for that object in the given situation. Thus, to construct free-body diagrams, it is extremely important to know the various types of forces. Therefore, the free body diagram of the ankle joint axis will have the forces to dorsiflex the tibia

and plantarflex the tibia since it is mainly a sagittal plane mover.

#447: What is the definition of a Couple of Forces? A couple of force will create a moment which will tend to make the object rotate.

#448: The coupling of forces acts in our complex world of biomechanics with every step. Imagine the pronatory forces which act on the subtalar joint coupled with the supinatory forces acting to resist this pronation. Describe the typical external forces created on a pronatory foot in podiatric biomechanics daily. Ground Reactive Force medial to the subtalar joint axis are supinatory. Orthotic Rx variables medial to the subtalar joint axis are supinatory. Shoe gear when high medial support can be supinatory. Taping can be done to apply only supinatory moments around the subtalar joint. Muscle strengthening can be done to isolate the muscles that supinate around the subtalar joint axis.

#449: Define a moment in physics in one sentence. A moment is the force to produce rotation. The moment of a force depends on the magnitude of the force and the distance from the axis of rotation.

#450: How would you explain how the subtalar joint is not in equilibrium when the heel is 14 degrees everted to the tibia bisection? The position of the subtalar joint is very pronated at this position. This gives mechanical power to the muscles which pronate the subtalar joint, and makes it very difficult for the supinators to work. The pronatory moments are far greater than the supinatory moments.

#451: Clinicians considering the forces exerted on the body in sports will begin to adapt their treatment to minimize overload affects. What are common treatment modalities that can help with this reduction of stress? Cross training more, taping, orthotics, changes in activity, elimination of high intensity activities too close together.

#452: Using the Rotational Equilibrium concept, what is the effect of shortening a lever arm to the rotational force (moment) created? The shorter the lever arm, the less the moment produced.

#453: When we think about patients with very pronated medially deviated feet, are the ground reactive forces barefoot generating more supinatory or pronatory moments? Pronatory

#454: The medially deviated subtalar joint axis provides a biomechanical challenge in applying appropriate force to help with the over pronation. What are 3 common techniques that accomplish that, and which one seems the most focused on the medial heel area? Varus wedging heel and forefoot, Inverted Technique, Medial Kirby Skive (most focused medial heel).

#455: Center of Pressure is a force plate analysis. If you had access to that information, how could CoP and Subtalar Axis position help in your orthotic designs?

If the CoP is lateral to the AST, the orthotic device must correct for pronation. If the CoP is medial to the AST, the orthotic device must correct for supination. If CoP is under AST, the orthotic device needs to be neutral balanced.

#456: There are various forces at play on the foot and rotatory forces having the ability to rotate structures around an axis are called what? And, how is it measured? Moments. Moments are measured by the magnitude of the force and the distance perpendicular to the axis it is acting on.

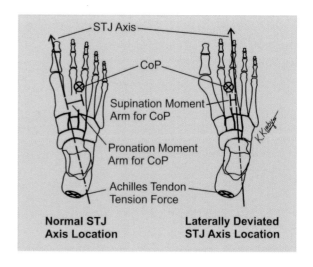

#457: From the illustration above, the achilles tendon is a natural supinator around the subtalar joint axis attaching medially to that axis. When in gait, does the achilles produce its most powerful subtalar joint supination? Middle to end of midstance

#458: The above implies that a medial deviated subtalar joint axis may not be a powerful pronatory force on the foot due to CoP. Please explain. For some feet, the medial deviated subtalar joint axis does not force the CoP medially, and the overall foot pronation is relatively mild.

#459: The development of a rocker bottom flatfoot (primarily in the sagittal plane) from an equinus tight achilles condition (primarily a sagittal plane deformity is a great example of this concept of planar dominance. What is a similar planar dominant problem at the knee also caused by equinus forces? Genu Recurvatum

Chapter 9

#460: As we begin to discuss Over Pronation Syndrome, what are the various types of over pronation treated (a wide range of answers are accepted)? Poor position left by pronatory problems, speed of pronation, lack of pronation for shock absorption, etc

#461: Using the Rule of 3, what are common biomechanical causes of tibial sesamoid stress that should be evaluated and treated if found? Excessive pronation with medial column overload, plantar flexed first metatarsal, hypomobile first ray, poor bone health

#462: Using the Rule of 3, what are common biomechanical causes of 4th metatarsal stress that should be evaluated and treated if found? Lateral overload from structural deformities leading to supination tendencies, activities that cause lateral overload, hypermobility in the 5th MCJ, and poor bone health.

#463: Using the Rule of 3, what are common biomechanical causes of peroneal tendon stress on the lateral ankle area that should be evaluated and treated if found? Structural deformities leading to abnormal supination tendencies, weak peroneals, and lateral ankle ligament instabilities

#464: What is a common example of pronation only occurring in late midstance? Pronation related to contact phase supination

#465: Many times this sport specific pronation is not seen in walking gait evaluation or indicated in their biomechanical examinations. What modification is essential in a custom insert for this problem? More pronation control in a sport specific orthotic device (only worn for that activity).

#466: What would you expect to see if a patient brought in 3 pairs of shoes (neutral, stability, and maximal control) and you could watch the same orthotic device in each? More pronation control from the orthotic device and shoe with the more stable the shoe. Perhaps even over correction in the maximal control and orthotic device.

#467: What would you expect to see if a patient brought in 3 pairs of shoes (all neutral but zero drop, moderate heel drop, and maximal heel drop) and you could watch the same orthotic device in each? More pronation in the zero drop shoes which make the athlete more flatfooted

#468: People have weak spots. Dr Blake uses a Rule of 3 to discover 2 other (and perhaps more) problems leading to an injury if over pronation is listed as one of the causes. What would be 2 other common causes of second metatarsal stress fracture? Structurally long 2nd metatarsal and hypermobile or dorsiflexed 1st metatarsal

#469: Remember to always make a patient more stable. What is the Stage of Bunion development that surgery should be at least considered? Stage 4

#470: Chronic overload of the 2nd MPJ due to over pronation can lead to what injuries? Second metatarsal stress fracture, second MPJ capsulitis, second MPJ plantar plate injuries

#471: Summarize in which situations why the motion of over pronation ends up hurting the 2nd metatarsal and not the first or just medial column. Over pronation is the source of global laxity in the foot. As weight moves from medial to lateral, the over mobility typically allows the first metatarsal to move dorsally trapping the stress on the 2nd metatarsal.

#472: How does a tight achilles tendon, which can cause abnormal pronation, also produce excessive pressure on the metatarsals leading to nerve hypersensitivity? A tight achilles tendon places plantigrade pressure on the metatarsal heads, which can stress the plantar soft tissues.The local nerves can then secondarily inflame in their protection mode.

#473: The plantar fascia is a tertiary support for our feet. Over pronation of the foot can cause instability of the primary ligaments, thus making the intrinsic muscles work harder. Theorize how this scenario could place stress on the plantar fascia especially if the intrinsic muscles were not strong. In an unstable foot, the weaker the muscles places the stress on the ligaments to support the foot.

#474: An unstable cuboid renders the peroneal longus tendon utterly useless. Explain why stabilizing the cuboid, even if it requires an Inverted Orthotic Device, can make the lateral ankle so much more stable. Stability of the cuboid anchors the peroneus longus allowing good propulsion with first metatarsal plantar flexion stabilizing the medial column. Also, a rock solid cuboid makes the lateral foot and lateral very stable.

#475: If there is an accessory navicular, when did it fully form and how much of the posterior tibial tendon attaches into it instead of the navicular bone? Accessory Naviculars fully form by 16 years old, and 10-80% approximately of the normal posterior tibial tendon attaches into it.

#476: If abnormal excessive pronation causes the foot to become a loose bag of bones (some more than others), which destabilizes the cuboid, how would you summarize its effects on the peroneus longus tendon, the first ray, and the lateral ankle? With an unstable cuboid, the peroneus longus can not plantar flex the first metatarsal needed for propulsion, therefore the first ray is unstable, and the lateral foot and ankle unstable. This is one reason ankle sprains can be indirectly caused by over pronation.

#477: What is the strongest muscle attaching into the tibia that decelerates subtalar joint pronation? Gastrocnemius has some tibial fibers, the soleus is mainly tibia and some fibula.

#478: The discussion above was on the stress to decelerate over pronation placed on the soleus. What are 2 common reasons found in our biomechanical examinations which analyze possible soleus weakness which would make it strain easier? AJDF knee bent shows a tight or over flexible soleus (both weakening), and the inability to do 12 bent knee single heel raises (gold standard of soleus strength)

#479: Over pronation of the foot compresses which side of the knee joint? Lateral

#480: Patellofemoral injuries was one of the first sports knee injuries that Podiatrists were treating with great success in the 1970s. Explain how the internal rotation of the limb increases the power of the vastus lateralis. As the femur internally rotates, the vastus lateralis is stretched, or placed in tone or tension, and the VL is also centered making the most powerful of the quadriceps 5 muscles.

#481: Flat feet has been proposed as a precursor to some ACL tears, since it

preloads the ligament as the foot abnormally pronates. If abnormal foot pronation places the knee more internal and flexed, why would that put stress on the ACL ligament? Pronation places the center of the knee more internal and forward placing the protection of falling forward into the hands of the ACL.

#482A: There are 2 medial and 2 lateral hamstrings. Please name them and explain why tight hamstrings strain easier than normal length hamstrings. Medial: Semimembranosis and Semitendinosis Lateral: Long and Short Head of Biceps Femoris.Tight muscle is harder to contract due to close proximity of the actin and myosin fibrils.

#482B: Name the 28 injuries or pain areas that can be caused or aggravated by over pronation. This implies that treatment of that over pronation may reduce or eliminate present symptoms.
1. First Metatarsal Phalangeal Joint Pain
2. Sesamoid Injuries
3. Bunions
4. Second Metatarsal Phalangeal Joint Capsulitis
5. Metatarsalgia
6. Second Metatarsal Stress Fractures
7. Morton's Neuroma or Neuritis
8. Hammertoes
9. Intrinsic Muscle Strain
10. Plantar Fasciitis
11. Anterior Tibial Tendonitis
12. Lateral sinus tarsitis
13. Cuboid Syndrome
14. Lateral Ankle Impingement

15. Posterior Tibial Injuries
16. Tarsal Tunnel Syndrome
17. Peroneus Longus Strain
18. Achilles Strain
19. Tibial Stress Fractures
20. Medial Soleus Strain
21. Lateral Knee Compartment Syndrome
22. Pes Anserinus Tendonitis/Bursitis
23. Patellofemoral Injuries
24. Anterior Cruciate Injuries
25. Medial Hamstring Strains
26. Iliotibial Band Syndrome
27. Piriformis Syndrome
28. Low Back Pain

#483: Lateral support in custom orthotic devices utilizing Root techniques comes from balancing forefoot valgus situations. What are the 3 common everted forefoot deformities that can lead to lateral foot overload and one main tibial problem producing the same lateral overload? Forefoot valgus, Plantarflexed First Ray, Forefoot Pronatus, Tibial Varum

#484: If excessive supination will shift weight more lateral in a foot, what are some reasons that the 4th metatarsal develops the overuse injury, not the 5th? Plantar flexed 4th metatarsal, hypermobile 5th metatarsal, gait pattern where weight goes through 4th more than 5th

#485: Cuboid pain can be produced by lateral overload. What 5 joint articulations could be involved? CC, C4thM, C5thM, C3rdM, and CN.

#486: How can lateral ankle instability produced by over supination cause medial ankle pain? Why in an acute inversion sprain is pain medially possibly indicative of something significant? The inversion of the talus on the tibial can cause injury to the medial ankle. With an inversion ankle sprain, the soft tissue gets injured laterally, but the bone can get injured medially.

#487: With the high cost of athletic shoes, patients can be prone to wearing them too long. When they begin to break down laterally, even in a patient with normal biomechanics, what types of ankle problems can they develop related to over supination? Peroneal strain of either tendon and medial ankle impingement symptoms.

#488: So many stress fractures (or full fractures) can occur by abnormal muscle contraction only. If a patient presents with lateral leg pain, why would it be important to differentiate the pain from bone pain versus peroneal muscle or tendon pain? You want to discover if there is a fibular stress fracture.

#489: What 2 very important structures attach into the head of the fibula? Lateral Collateral Ligament and Lateral Hamstrings

#490: How could over tightness of the lateral hamstring lead to proximal tib-fib symptoms? The lateral hamstrings attach into the head of the fibula and can cause irritation across the tib-fib joint when it pulls too hard.

#491: What side of the knee is compressed when you supinate the foot? Medial

#492: Would a patient with a higher than normal Q Angle be more likely to get iliotibial band syndrome while running? A high Q Angle means that there is more deformity at the knee for the muscles and ligaments to attempt to stabilize. Also, a high Q Angle typically means more internal rotation of the tibia on the femur irritating the IT Band.

#493: For shock absorption problems in the lower leg, the Hannaford custom orthotic device, primarily discussed in the next book, is ideal. What is the type of material a Hannaford is made out of, and can you also correct for pronation or supination? Plastazote® material in layers, and corrections can be made for varus or valgus.

#494: As the SI joint moves inferiorly, it also moves in what direction? When palpating the ASIS during lower extremity limb length exam, if you find the right ASIS to be forward to the left, what does that mean? The SI joint moves anterior and inferior, or the opposite. The anterior position of the ASIS right to left signifies a pelvic tilt.

#495: What are the seven Rxs for orthotic laboratories based on the pronation to supination spectrum? Root Balanced, Mild Anti-Supination Modifications, Moderate Anti-Supination Modifications, 3-4 Degree Varus Anti-Pronation Modifications, 5-7 Degree Varus Anti-Pronation Modifications, Over 7 Varus Anti-Pronation Modifications, PTTD Anti-Pronation Modifications

Chapter 10

#496: What are 7 common gait signs of a leg length difference? Head tilt, shoulder drop, asymmetrical arm swing, dominance to one side, uneven belt line, asymmetrical lower extremity motion, possible hip hike

#497: Explain why a runner with a short leg would do better with a full length lift versus a heel lift while running hills. Hill running typically requires the athlete to be on the ball of their feet the majority of the time.

#498: If a patient has chronic low back pain for years, and you have measured around one half inch short right side, how would you get them into lift therapy smartly? Start Low and Go Slow is the mantra with lift therapy. Every 2 weeks increase ⅛ inch, and start with one eighth inch.

#499: There are pros and cons with using heel lifts vs full length lifts. What would the obvious choice be in a runner? Since runners are always up onto the ball of their feet, full length lifts make more sense.

#500: When one side is more pronated, orthotic Rxs can be to correct for the asymmetry or avoid it. If a long leg pronates more, and the orthotic correction is more support on that side, what is this doing to the asymmetry of the long leg? You are making the long leg even longer which may have to happen. You have to decide it is better to treat the limb length or the pronation first.

#501: If a patient is walking, and their left side is more unstable than their right, and they are left handed, what could that mean (many answers)? In a left handed person, the right side is their more stable supportive side, so this is pretty normal.

#502: If you measure a short right leg on the more pronated side, what are the possibilities? This happens 20% of the time. The limb length discrepancy should be measured with both feet in subtalar joint neutral, or at least in the orthotic devices that they will be wearing. If the short leg is more pronated, there may not be any structural limb length difference, only functional.

#503: If you measure a short right leg, but the left leg is more pronated, what are the possibilities? The longer left leg is pronating to compensate and may be longer than measured. This speaks to a functional component to this limb length discrepancy.

Chapter 11

#504: Why are we taught not to stretch through pain? Pain will cause the muscle to tighten up for protection, and the muscle is tighter after the painful stretch.

#505: What are two ways to measure gastrocnemius strength? Hint: One is related to flexibility. Ability to do straight knee single heel raise, and measuring flexibility

to evaluate for over tightness or over flexibility.

#506: Explain the basic principle of Contract Relax self application. You contract the muscle to warm up and fatigue, then stretch it, and repeat multiple times. This is found to stretch muscles better than normal stretching.

#507: What is most difficult to do for a patient right after they are injured: isotonic or isometric exercises? Isotonic since it is unknown how much they can do, so it is easy to put on too much weight.

#508: What is a benchmark for strengthening and how is it established for a patient with resistance bands? A benchmark establishes the amount of strength a patient can do at a certain day, and is used to mark progress. For example, May 1st the patient could do 2 sets of 15 with Level 2 resistance bands, but July 1st 2 sets of 20 with Level 4.

#509: As an injury gets better, rehabilitation procedures must allow some pain to enter the equation. What does it mean when an athlete is allowed to participate as long as the pain is back to normal in 2 days? This is typically reserved for the Return to Activity Phase when we are doing activities that are putting more and more stress on the injured tissue.

#510A: Why is lower extremity evening strengthening preferred? If you fatigue while doing them, you will soon go to bed and not have to walk around on fatigued muscles during the day.

#510B: What are the 8-9 top muscles to strenghten to slow down the foot pronation? Foot Intrinsics, Posterior Tibial, Anterior Tibial, Peroneus Longus, Gastrocnemius, Soleus, Lateral Hamstring, Sartorius, External Hip Rotators, Iliopsoas.

#511: With the 6 main ankle motions, what muscle is strengthened with each? Achilles complex with plantarflexion, Peroneus Longus with Eversion Ankle Neutral, Peroneus Brevis with Eversion Ankle Plantarflexed, Posterior Tibial with Inversion Ankle Plantarflexed, Anterior Tibial with Inversion Ankle Dorsiflexed, Extensors with Dorsiflexion.

#512: Explain how to do AROM dorsiflexion exercises without and with gravity. With gravity you pull up your foot towards the ceiling, with your foot perpendicular to the ground. Without gravity, you are doing the same pull, but your foot is parallel to the ground.

#513: After level 4 two sets of 20 repetitions, what would the next progression be of resistance band? 1 set of 25 reps followed by 1 set of 20 reps.

#514: If you are doing 2 sets of a resistance band, how much time should be between each set to rest? Around 1 minute at least.

#515: Doing a single leg press for patellofemoral joint pain patients, should your foot be straight or turned out slightly? Slightly turned out to help activate the vastus medialis.

#516: Following an achilles rupture and successful surgery or cast immobilization, what must be assumed in terms of the overall achilles tendon strength the first day of rehab? Zero strength exists

#517: What is one reason due to muscle strength that we place ankle sprains in an ankle brace for a while? After an ankle sprain, our muscles shut down due to pain initially, and then weaken with immobilization.This makes us very prone to another sprain until the muscles are restrengthened.

#518: In evaluating foot function, a patient was found to have poor FHL tone. What spinal disc could be involved? L3/L4

Chapter 12

#519: Poor Shock Absorption can be part of a patient's intrinsic biomechanics, or just part of the mechanics of their activity. Discuss prolonged downhill running as a cause of poor shock absorption. When you run normally you have to absorb 2-3 times your bodyweight at impact and 5-7 times your bodyweight running downhill.

#520: What blood test should always be taken when a patient presents with an overuse related stress fracture related to poor shock absorption? Vitamin D

#521: How does an osteopenic bone density make you more prone for a stress fracture with high impact loads? The lower your bone health is, the earlier the bone will fatigue and cause injury.

#522: I learned years ago that a hard piece of plastic can be an incredible source of shock absorption? Explain how a plastic orthotic device can help absorb shock in a runner. Ground reactive force exerts shock at impact with ground and that force is dissipated by anything running perpendicular.

#523: In the orthotic/shoe world, if you have a very unstable shoe, the orthotic will help gain some stability. What type of orthotic device would you need in a very stable hard shoes like the Brooks Beast in a patient with chronic tibial stress fractures/reactions? Some to minimum support, but high on shock absorption. Have your lab make their version of a Hannaford device.

#524A: Why can it make a big difference for a runner to run the downhill part of a course first instead of at the end (in terms of the development of stress fractures)? Muscles protect bones and muscles are typically better at the beginning of a run before they get exhausted.

#524B: What are several possible ways that a runner can decrease the shock stress to the legs if vulnerable for stress fractures? Avoid downhills, slow pace down, softer shoes, orthotic devices, less rear foot strike pattern.

#525: What are 7 common causes of lateral instability in patients that can cause

problems? Ankle ligament damage, peroneus brevis weakness, peroneus longus weakness, everted forefoot deformities, high rearfoot varus deformities, ligamentous laxity, broken down shoes, etc.

#526: What does a simple varus wedge at the foot do to the knee alignment in a patient with excessive internal femoral rotation? The varus wedge decreases the internal positioning, or slows down the internal rotation, of the knee.

#527: Medial Knee Compartment problems are typically extension issues, and Lateral Knee Compartment problems are typically flexion issues. Explain why keeping the knee slightly flexed can help medial knee joint line pain. Keeping the patient functioning with soft knees can decrease the compression forces across the joint caused by full extension.

#528: Gait evaluation can be a key to discovering abnormalities years before symptoms. What problems may be associated with the gait finding of Hip Hike? Long Leg or Arthritic Hip or Hip Replacement

Index

Supination Problems 638
Supination, Shoe Recommendations 567
Supination Syndrome 637-45
Synergy of Flexing 598

T

Tailor's Bunion 639
Talar Mobilization 496
TallMenShoes.com 494
Taping, Achilles 499-500, 515
Taping, Ilio-Tibial Band 566, 635
Taping, Inversion Control, Leukotape 503-504, 509, 534-5
Taping Knee 538-9, 555, 563
Tarsal Tunnel Syndrome 631
Tennis Leg 516
Tib-Fib Sprain, Proximal 642
Tibial Stress Fractures 527-31, 632
Tibial Stress Fractures, locations 527
Tissue Stress 603-6

U

Upper Hamstring Strain 576-580

V

Valgus Wedges 506, 533, 546
Varus Wedge 542, 547, 550-1, 556, 569, 589-90
Varus Wedge Forefoot Striker 556
Vastus Lateralis Stretch 540-1
Vitamin D 568

W

Weak Link in the Chain 620
Wedged Shoes 529
Weed, Dr John 609
Widen Base of Gait 537

X

Xray Anterior Ankle Spurs 492
Xray Standing AP Pelvis 572, 588, 654

Z

Zero Drop Shoes 495, 513, 579